Advanced
EXERCISES IN DIAGNOSTIC RADIOLOGY

16

BLUNT AND PENETRATING TRAUMA

ALLAN E. FISCH, M.D.
Assistant Chief of Radiology,
Department of Radiology,
Mount Zion Hospital, San Francisco;
Clinical Instructor of Radiology,
University of California, San Francisco

HELEN C. REDMAN, M.D.
Associate Chief of Radiology,
Mount Zion Hospital, San Francisco;
Clinical Associate Professor of Radiology,
Stanford University and University of
California, San Francisco

W. B. SAUNDERS COMPANY • 1982

PHILADELPHIA • LONDON • TORONTO • MEXICO CITY • RIO DE JANEIRO • SYDNEY • TOKYO

W. B. Saunders Company:　West Washington Square
Philadelphia, PA　19105

1 St. Anne's Road
Eastbourne, East Sussex BN21 3UN, England

1 Goldthorne Avenue
Toronto, Ontario M8Z 5T9, Canada

Apartado 26370 — Cedro 512
Mexico 4, D.F., Mexico

Rua Coronel Cabrita, 8
Sao Cristovao Caixa Postal 21176
Rio de Janeiro, Brazil

9 Waltham Street
Artarmon, N.S.W. 2064, Australia

Ichibancho, Central Bldg., 22-1 Ichibancho
Chiyoda-Ku, Tokyo 102, Japan

Library of Congress Cataloging in Publication Data

Fisch, Allan E.

Blunt and penetrating trauma.

(Advanced exercises in diagnostic radiology; 16)

1. Wounds　and　injuries — Diagnosis.　2. Diagnosis, Radi-
oscopic.　I. Redman, Helen C.　II. Title.　III. Series
[DNLM: 1. Wounds and injuries — Radiography.
2. Wounds, Penetrating — Radiography.

W1 AD 402E v.16/WO 700 F528b]

RC78.E89 vol. 16 [RD93.7]　　616.07′57s　　82-47575

ISBN 0-7216-3677-2　　[617′.10757]　　AACR2

BLUNT AND PENETRATING TRAUMA

Advanced Exercises in Diagnostic Radiology — 16 　　　　ISBN　0-7216-3677-2

Last digit is the print number:　　9　8　7　6　5　4　3　2　1

PREFACE

Soft tissue trauma takes many forms, some of which require radiologic evaluation for proper management. The radiologist is well versed in the procedures that he can perform and their limitations and their interpretation; the referring physician knows the questions that need answers in a specific patient; but each is less familiar with the methods and problems of the other. This volume illustrates a variety of problems associated with soft tissue trauma and tries to demonstrate the radiographic approaches available for solving them. If you gain nothing else from this book, the importance of communication among the physicians treating injured patients should stay with you. Only with communication and cooperation among physicians can the patients receive the optimum diagnostic and therapeutic measures.

The book has six chapters. The first one is an introductory chapter defining soft tissue trauma as it will be used in this volume and discussing the variety of radiologic examinations generally available. The demands that these procedures make on patients are described, as are the requirements for a successful examination. The remaining chapters deal with areas of the body loosely grouped by organ system. A variety of injuries are discussed in each chapter, and the assorted radiologic procedures used in their evaluation are illustrated. We have tried to demonstrate that many problems can be approached in several ways and to indicate reasons for choosing one method over another in a specific patient. Sometimes only a single "correct" approach to a given problem is illustrated, but in other situations a variety of technics are presented. The reader should try to learn the variety of tests available along with their strengths and weaknesses so that when he is faced with a clinical problem he will be able to choose the best approach for his patient.

The cases each include one or more related clinical problems. While the injuries suffered by each patient are those that are illustrated, we have invented almost all the situations in which the injury occurred both to provide anonymity for the actual patient and to present a situation in which such an injury typically happens. The procedures illustrated were actually performed in each patient but not necessarily for the reasons given or in the sequence that we illustrate. Again, this rearranging is done to make one or more teaching points and should be considered in that light.

The book may be approached as a whole or by chapters or by case group. Related injuries are grouped together, and while the progression of cases within a chapter follows a reasoned sequence, most will stand on their own. Though we hope the cases will hold the reader's interest, it is more important that the reader come away with the concept of flexibility in dealing with the injured patient and that he gain a fuller understanding of the many radiological procedures that may help in diagnosis of the patient.

ACKNOWLEDGMENTS

Completion of this book, or in fact any radiologic text, is made possible by the cooperation and assistance of many people. Within our department, our colleagues have provided interesting case material and put up with our abstraction. Technologists have taken that "extra-beautiful" radiograph for publication. Probably most important, Melanie Liszka has typed, retyped, made editorial suggestions and again retyped our manuscript. Without her it would have never reached completion.

After searching through our files we were still in need of good illustrative material. This was willingly provided by a long list of past residents and colleagues in other hospitals. Specifically, we would like to thank Dr. James Waskey at the Kaiser Permanente Hospital in Oakland, California, for the case material used in illustrations 2–2t, 2–2u, 2–11e, 2–11f, 3–6a, 3–6b, 3–10a, 3–10b, 3–13a, 3–13b, 3–15, 3–17b, 3–17c, 3–18a, 3–18b, 3–18c, 4–2d, 4–3e, 4–6l, 4–6m, 4–6n, 5–1a, 5–1e, 5–1f, 5–2g, 5–2h, 5–2i, 5–2j, 5–3a, 5–3b, 5–4d, 5–4e, 5–4f, 6–2, 6–5a, 6–5b and 6–14. Dr. Joy Price from Herrick Hospital in Oakland, California, provided the case material used in illustrations 2–9c, 4–5c, 4–5f, 4–5g, 4–5h, 4–5i and 4–5j. Dr. Susan M. Gootnick of the San Francisco United States Public Health Service Hospital provided us with illustrations used for cases 4–7 and 4–9, which ended quite a search. Dr. David Soffa of San Francisco loaned us the material for 3–1a and 3–1b. Two Stanford colleagues also came to our aid. Dr. Henry Jones provided illustrations 5–5a, 5–5b and 5–5c. Dr. Lewis Wexler gave us 3–9a and 3–9b. Dr. J. Walters of the Palo Alto Clinic provided the remainder of that case, 3–9c, 3–9d and 3–9e. The group at San Francisco General Hospital provided us with the material for Case 2–6. Dr. Richard Wolfe of our group permitted us to use the arthrogram illustrated in Case 6–7. Last, but not least, Dr. Erick Lang of Louisiana State University provided us with the material used in 5–4a, 5–4b and 5–4c. Without the cooperation of these colleagues in sending us good case material or letting us search their files, we would not have been able to complete this project.

We received assistance from Drs. Y. M. Ting and S. R. Reuter, who gave us permission to use illustrations 4–3a, 4–3b, 4–4a and 4–4c, which were published in an article entitled "Hollow Viscus Injury in Blunt Abdominal Trauma," *American Journal of Roentgenology*, Volume *119*, page 408, 1973. Dr. Ting provided us with the films from her teaching file.

The American Medical Association has also given us permission to use illustrations 6–11 and 6–13, which were originally published in an article by Helen C. Redman, M.D., entitled, "Thoracic, Abdominal and Peripheral Trauma: Evaluation with Angiography," in the *Journal of the American Medical Association*, Volume 237, pages 2415–2418, May 30, 1977; Copyright 1977, American Medical Association.

Finally, we thank our respective families for their tolerance of our endeavor and for their moral support during these months of creation.

TABLE OF CONTENTS

Preface

Acknowledgments

INTRODUCTION

In this exercise we have used a broad definition of "trauma" to encompass the spectrum of problems encountered in the practice of acute care medicine. It is obvious that the unfortunate person who is struck by a car has been injured, but toxic chemicals and even innocent household objects can also cause serious damage when they are misused. Most patients with fractures have associated soft tissue trauma. These injuries are often minor but can threaten life or limb when there is vascular impairment or a cervical spinal cord contusion, for example. The barefoot child who steps on a sewing needle has a penetrating soft tissue injury and frequently has a retained foreign body that must be extracted. The rather commonplace 'concussion' is really a contusion of the brain and may include hemorrhage. A similar blow to the head can lead to more significant injury such as a subdural hematoma. Aspiration of gasoline while siphoning it from one tank to another can cause both pulmonary and gastric damage. Therapeutic or diagnostic procedures often traumatize normal tissues and may have serious sequelae. Patients with any of these problems may come to an emergency room, office or clinic for acute care or may be seen during the evolution of their trauma-related disease.

Blunt trauma is more common than penetrating injury in most nonmilitary practices. By definition it is a closed injury, though there may be associated penetrating injury. Blunt trauma commonly occurs in motor vehicle accidents, falls, brawls and childhood pranks. The actual incident may seem minor, but the consequences can be major and symptoms can be delayed days or weeks. The child who falls off his bike, hitting the handlebars as he tumbles, inspects his skinned knee, rubs his side, wipes his tears and rides off may have injured his spleen or kidney but will begin to complain hours or days later. Everyone has had a blow to the head at one time or another; now and then chronic headaches or neurologic impairment after such an injury signals the development of a subdural hematoma. Deceleration injuries most frequently occur in head-on automobile accidents. Drivers are especially vulnerable, since they often hit the steering wheel. Rapid deceleration can lead to aortic laceration, a frequently rapidly fatal injury, which can sometimes be repaired by prompt surgical intervention. While the solid abdominal and retroperitoneal organs are more frequently injured by blunt trauma than the hollow ones, the bowel can be contused, develop hematomas, or actually rupture. Radiology often plays a significant role in the diagnosis of such blunt injuries.

There are two major categories of penetrating injury. The first is the low velocity penetrating injury. Stab wounds are a good example of low velocity trauma. The injury can be minor or serious depending on the site of the stab wound and depth of penetration. There is little tissue damage at any distance from the actual path of the wound, so that if surgical exploration is warranted, it can be confined to the path of injury itself. The role of radiology in these patients is usually limited, but can be important when there is a pneumothorax, vascular damage or other serious injury.

High velocity penetrating wounds are most common in warfare, but civilians are now more frequently at risk. These are best characterized by the wound caused by a bullet travelling at high speed. The hallmark of such trauma is the blast injury that surrounds the path of the missile. The severity of the blast injury varies with the tissues traversed and with the size, shape and speed of the missile involved. While these patients will have surgery almost without exception, x-rays may be requested to determine the extent of the injury. Such films may be needed only to demonstrate associated fractures or the location of the missile, or may be more complicated, including angiography or other special procedures. Any radiographic study in these patients must be tailored to the individual situation and should be done expeditiously.

There are a variety of injuries that are neither blunt nor penetrating in nature. Inhalation of toxic substances, aspiration or ingestion of acid and swallowing or aspiration of foreign bodies are all examples. There is also the large class of iatrogenic trauma, including arteriovenous fistulae after liver biopsy, pseudo-aneurysms after arterial catheterization, esophageal perforation during endoscopy and adverse drug reactions. Some are obvious immediately, while others may take some time to become symptomatic.

Each patient who has been injured should be given individualized care. Injuries are highly varied and are rarely as predictable as other illnesses. Invariably, radiographic evaluation will need to be fitted to the specific situation and should not be allowed to fall into a "routine." For example: depth of depression of skull fragments must be determined from film tangential to the fracture or from a CT scan. This information can seldom be obtained from the routine skull series, and the technologist must be directed to position the patient accordingly. A broken sewing needle in a thigh must be located by x-ray in a fashion that will allow a successful removal without an extensive surgical exploration of the subcutaneous tissues. This may require fluoroscopy or radiopaque markers. The need for skilled radiologic consultation is always important, but especially in more serious injuries the radiologist, the referring physicians and the technologist should all become involved in obtaining the most useful films and special studies.

Care must be taken not to aggravate the injuries that are present. For example, when a patient is admitted with a deceleration injury and there is clinical suspicion of both a lacerated aorta and a cervical spine fracture, the patient's neck must be immobilized until the spine is satisfactorily evaluated. A supine chest film will be all that can be obtained prior to anteroposterior and cross-table lateral cervical spine films. In the seriously injured patient, speed in diagnosis becomes paramount and all those involved with the patient must remember that the primary goal is to get the appropriate therapy under way in the proper sequence. It should be clear that if you have a patient who is rapidly losing consciousness from an epidural hematoma shown on a CT scan, you should not bother to x-ray a possible extremity fracture on the way to surgery, but simply immobilize the part. Once the epidural hematoma has been taken care of, possible broken bones can be investigated. When two life-threatening injuries coexist, a decision must be made about which to approach first. Errors may occur in these judgments, but you cannot afford to waste time speculating on the proper approach. Perhaps a true case history will best illustrate these points.

Mr. M. V. A. was flagged down on the Interstate by the police because he had no rear license plate. When he walked behind his car to look, he was struck by another car travelling at an estimated 45 mph. He was knocked forcefully forward onto the trunk of his own car and his legs were pinned between his car and the one that hit him. The policeman immediately called an ambulance, which arrived in about five minutes. The ambulance attendant called the emergency room, saying that while Mr. M. V. A. was conscious when they got to him, he was no longer so and had a very weak, thready pulse, a rapidly expanding abdomen, two obviously broken legs and large bruises over his chest, face and head. The driver estimated their arrival time at the hospital as three minutes. They had started one intravenous line, were giving oxygen nasally and were trying to start a second intravenous line. (You have about three minutes to assemble the proper team and have a tentative treatment plan in mind. Does this patient need x-rays? Now or later?)

Mr. M. V. A. is met at the ambulance entrance; the second I.V. is running. He is non-responsive and does have a very tense abdomen. You think you feel a carotid pulse. The patient is taken straight to the operating room with a diagnosis of massive intra-abdominal hemorrhage. This decision is correct; about six feet of small bowel have been stripped from the mesentery and the abdomen is filled with blood. Control of the hemorrhage goes well, the appropriate small bowel is resected and the abdomen explored for other injuries. None are found. With this problem under control and with pulse and blood pressure obtainable there is time to think about the patient's other known and unknown injuries.

Starting with the head, Mr. M. V. A. had a severe blow to his forehead and lost consciousness quite rapdily, and the anesthesiologist says his pupils are unequal. He probably has a significant head injury. His cardiac and respiratory status are stable now that blood volume is being restored, but this does not exclude a significant thoracic injury. An orthopedic consultant is concerned about the vascular supply to the left leg.

X-rays are now in order. While the patient is still under anesthesia AP and lateral skull films are taken and show a linear skull fracture. The supine chest has many of the hallmarks of aortic laceration. Both femurs are fractured and there is rotatory dislocation of the left knee. (What do you do now?)

Angiography is chosen as the single modality that could answer the several questions that are raised. Mr. M. V. A. is about 30 years old, so that procedure is technically simple. A thoracic aortogram demonstrates a typical aortic laceration just distal to the left subclavian artery. Cerebral angiography demonstrates an epidural hematoma. Runoff filming shows that the vascular supply in the right leg is intact, but that there is a popliteal artery occlusion on the left.

The neurosurgeon, cardiac surgeon and orthopedist decide to approach the problems by first fixing the aorta, then evacuating the epidural hematoma and finally attempting to fix the left popliteal artery and reducing the femoral fractures. After 17 hours, Mr. M. V. A. is taken to the recovery room. The left popliteal artery repair is unsuccessful and amputation is performed on his third hospital day. Otherwise, his recovery is uneventful and he leaves the hospital 19 days later.

Mr. M. V. A. is a dramatic example of extensive injury, and he illustrates well the need for speed and flexibility in the evaluation and care of such patients. The physicians faced with trauma must be able to meet these demands on the one hand, and also fill the needs of the more frequent patient with lesser injuries. At the same time both the clinician and the radiologist must remember that much soft tissue trauma does not require radiologic assistance. As with all x-rays, you should be sure that films offer a reasonable chance of providing information that will be of use to you and the patient.

RADIOGRAPHIC TECHNIQUES

Among the considerations in choosing a diagnostic approach to an injured patient are the demands that a given procedure will make upon that patient. The length of time the procedure takes and the degree of patient cooperation required are two important factors. Some examinations have an intrinsic risk that must also be considered. Some procedures can be performed using a portable radiographic unit, while others require fluoroscopy or very specialized equipment to which the patient must be moved. This section describes in general terms the demands the various types of radiographic procedures make upon patients. These general factors should help you decide which examinations to choose in a given patient and also in what sequence to do them.

Plain Films

Simple x-rays of the extremities, chest or abdomen require relatively little patient cooperation and only a short time for each film. Aside from the hazards of moving and positioning some patients, plain films carry very little risk. While some soft tissue injuries such as pneumothorax and radiopaque foreign bodies are best studied with plain films, most soft tissue trauma is poorly, or incompletely, evaluated by such films. This is in contrast to bony trauma, which is generally best evaluated by plain films. Many plain films can be taken with a portable unit if necessary. The information obtained, however, is likely to be more limited than that obtained in a fixed radiographic installation.

Oral Contrast Medium Studies

These studies all should be done under fluoroscopic control, unless there is great difficulty or danger in moving the patient. Lack of fluoroscopic control and spot filming capability will greatly limit the usefulness of these techniques, but they may be occasionally performed on a "portable" basis. Either water soluble contrast material or a barium suspension can be used, depending on the problem. As a rule, when perforation is a concern, water soluble contrast material is preferable unless aspiration is a likely possibility. Studies of the esophagus are most satisfactory when the patient can drink on his own, but studies of the esophagus, stomach, duodenum and small bowel can all be performed through properly placed tubes when necessary. These studies rarely take less than 15 minutes and can be much more lengthy if the patient is difficult to position. Small bowel studies depend on peristalsis and may take hours when a paralytic ileus is present.

Barium will interfere with ultrasound, computed tomography, excretory urography and angiography. The sound beam used for an ultrasound will not pass through barium, and the very dense nature of barium obscures information and creates artifacts on computed tomography. Water soluble contrast material will interfere significantly less with ultrasound, but the concentration used for gastrointestinal studies may also interfere with CT scanning. Contrast material in the gastrointestinal tract will also obscure the kidneys and make visceral angiography difficult or impossible. Therefore, if you may need any of these examinations, they should precede oral contrast studies.

Contrast Studies Per Rectum

Barium or water soluble contrast material enemas must be done under fluoroscopic control. In the cooperative patient, a complete study rarely takes less than 15 minutes and can take considerably longer if the patient is unable to move easily. Fecal matter will degrade colon examinations, but this is generally not important under emergency conditions. These studies are more stressful to the patient than upper gastrointestinal examinations and can cause cardiac arrhythmias. If both lower and upper gastrointestinal studies are required, it is generally preferable to do the enema first. The contrast material will also interfere with ultrasound, CT, excretory urography and angiography so these studies should be performed first, if needed.

Studies Using Intravenous Contrast Material

The primary examination in this group is the excretory urogram. This study can be modified to meet the problem at hand and can take as little as 10 minutes. While it can be done with a portable unit, the study is much better performed by a fixed installation. While dehydration, poor renal function and previous serious contrast medium reaction are relative contraindications to urography, in the face of serious trauma these risks may be acceptable. The study requires very little patient cooperation except the ability to hold still. The exception to this is when a voiding study is requested following urography. Patient cooperation is mandatory for this procedure. As discussed, barium studies will interfere with urographic examinations, so these studies should be done first.

Ultrasound

An ultrasound examination cannot be performed through bone, air or barium. A profound ileus will make much of the abdomen impenetrable to this modality. In a non-emergency situation, abdominal studies are scheduled after the patient has been NPO for 6 to 12 hours. In the acutely injured patient, this may not be practical. Pelvic studies are most successful when the urinary bladder is distended. Since this can be accomplished by catheterization, the bladder can be distended rapidly in most patients when necessary.

Ultrasound studies carry no risk to the patient and require only minimal cooperation beyond the ability to hold still and briefly suspend respiration. Evaluation of the liver and spleen is improved by a good inspiratory effort, which is sometimes difficult for the injured patient. In addition, the ultrasound transducer must be pressed firmly on the area being scanned, and this maneuver can be quite painful in the presence of rib fractures or other injuries. If there is a skin wound over the area of concern, the examination may be limited or impossible to perform.

Ultrasound studies are variable in length but seldom take less than 20 minutes. Some portable ultrasound units are available primarily for real-time or dynamic scanning. Most studies will require transport of the patient to an ultrasound unit.

Computerized Tomography (CT)

Computerized tomography of the head requires that the patient be able to lie absolutely still for the duration of a scan, generally less than 10 seconds with the newer scanners. Aside from radiation, which is at an acceptable level, there is no risk to the patient with a non-contrast medium scan and only a slight risk of contrast medium reaction with a contrast-enhanced examination. An examination can be performed in less than 10 minutes once the patient has been placed in the scanner, and most units demonstrate the sections as they are completed so that a diagnosis can be made rapidly in injuries such as an epidural hematoma.

CT scans of the remainder of the body also require that the patient hold still. When the thorax or abdomen is being scanned, the ability to stop breathing for the duration of the scan will significantly improve resolution. Studies of the abdomen should be performed before any barium or concentrated water soluble contrast material is given, since these dense substances can obscure important information. It may be useful to give dilute oral contrast medium or intravenous contrast material to some patients, depending on the problem presented. CT body examinations are variable in length, depending upon the individual situation, but will rarely take less than 10 minutes.

Isotopic Examinations

The role of nuclear radiology in acute trauma is somewhat limited, but there are a variety of techniques that can be exceedingly useful, for example, liver or spleen scanning. While portable examinations can be performed if the equipment is available, the patient is generally required to go to the scanning area and to lie still for a varying length of time depending on the examination.

These examinations do not interfere with other radiographic examinations, nor do they carry any risk to the patient beyond the radiation exposure required to perform the test.

Special Studies

There are many special studies that can be used in trauma patients. Some are quite simple, such as injection of an abdominal stab wound track, retrograde urethrogram or cystogram. Others are more complicated, such as myelography or angiography. Most will be performed either by or with a radiologist. Many of these procedures can be performed on a portable basis, but this is not good practice. The best results are obtained in specially designed radiographic rooms, with fluoroscopic monitoring and skilled personnel. Portable examinations will produce a limited amount of information at greater risk to the patient because of inadequate controls in a bedside setting. Many special studies do have a definable complication rate, but usually the risk is more than met by the benefits expected. Though these procedures tend to be somewhat complex, they generally require little patient cooperation beyond the ability to lie reasonably still for a short period of time.

When it is likely that an acutely injured patient will need an emergency special study, consultation with the radiologist early during evaluation of the patient will be important in the diagnostic process. Radiologists are fully conversant with the requirements and benefits of these procedures and can help with the choice of appropriate studies, and initiate the preliminary preparations for the examination so that it is performed expeditiously.

The following chapters will illustrate blunt and penetrating trauma to various areas of the body. As you read the case histories, think how you might handle the problem. Try to assess the degree of urgency and make a plan of action. There are often several ways to approach these problems, so though you may differ in your approach from what was done in the case, you may still be dealing with the situation in an efficient and logical fashion. Your plan will be influenced by the equipment and personnel you have available. We have tried to indicate alternate techniques when reasonable, and in view of the rapidly changing radiologic technology, new approaches to trauma will always be appearing which will challenge current procedures for a position in the diagnosis of trauma.

CENTRAL NERVOUS SYSTEM, HEAD AND NECK

It is difficult to isolate bony from soft tissue trauma in the central nervous system and face because of the protective and supportive nature of the skull and facial bones. While it is the soft tissue component of the injury that is generally most important to the long-term health of the injured person, bony injury will play a greater role in this chapter than in most of the remaining sections of the book. The nature and location of a fracture will often be of use in determining what studies should be undertaken to evaluate the related soft tissue trauma. Pressure on the brain or spinal cord can cause irreversible damage very quickly, making it important to diagnose injuries such as depressed skull fractures, epidural and subdural hematomas and intramedullary hematomas rapidly so that appropriate therapy can be instituted. Care must be taken during the diagnostic evaluation not to jeopardize the patient or make an injury worse. A classic example is stabilization of the neck in suspected fracture or dislocation of the cervical spine. The aim is to avoid trauma to the cervical spinal cord. In the presence of a head injury the patient will need careful observation while undergoing a CT scan or other radiographic procedures.

The development of CT scanning has made an incredible difference in the diagnostic approach to head trauma. The skull series for fracture has a markedly diminished importance, since CT can demonstrate the degree of depression of bony fragments as well as the epidural and subdural hematomas, intracerebral bleeds and contusions. Identification of linear skull fractures is generally of much less clinical importance, and absence of such a fracture does not exclude intracranial pathology. In addition, isotopic brain scan for trauma is rarely needed, and cerebral angiography is seldom indicated, unless vascular injury is suspected. CT is faster, simpler, safer and more informative in many situations than use of all three other modalities. Of all the tests mentioned, only CT allows direct visualization of the parenchyma of the brain.

Non-neurologic soft tissue trauma to the head and neck that requires radiologic evaluation is less common. It has been included in this chapter because of anatomic proximity and because such injuries are sometimes associated with trauma involving the central nervous system. However, these injuries also include trauma to the larynx, trachea and esophagus, for example, which require an entirely different train of thought. Since flexibility is requisite to adequate diagnosis and care of injured patients, you should find this a useful exercise.

CASE 2–1:

BABIES B. C., A. J. AND B.W.

The three infants in this case illustrate trauma caused by vaginal delivery. These injuries are usually more dramatic than serious, but it is important to be familiar with them, since new parents are rarely fully rational about the health and welfare of their infant. Generally, these injuries occur with prolonged or difficult labor, especially one that has been mechanically assisted. No therapy is indicated for the swelling itself, but reassurance of the anxious family can be quite therapeutic.

When labor became prolonged and there were signs of fetal distress, B. C.'s mother was moved from the Alternate Birth Center to the delivery suite. A vaginal delivery was completed with the aid of forceps. B. C. has a good Apgar score but has marked swelling of the left side of his head. The parents still desire an early discharge, so skull films are taken to exclude significant injury to the skull. A lateral and a Towne view are illustrated. What do you see?

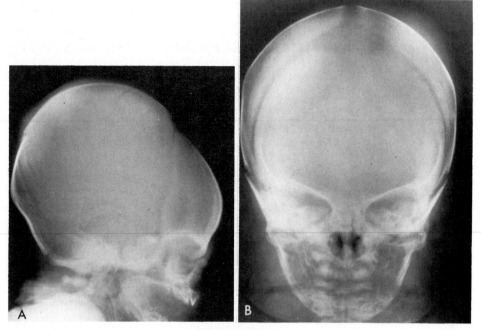

Figure 2–1a, b

There is a short non-depressed fracture of the left parietal bone. It extends from the sagittal suture and is best seen on the lateral film. More impressive is the soft tissue swelling over the left parietal bone. This is typical of a cephalhematoma, which is subperiosteal bleeding caused by birth trauma. Because of the subperiosteal location of the bleeding, the hematoma is confined to a single bone of the skull. B. C.'s parents are relieved and go home with their new baby the following day.

A. J.'s parents, on the other hand, arrive unexpectedly in your office when A. J. is 20 days old. They feel a hard mass on the left side of the head and are sure something is terribly wrong with their baby. A. J. is crying lustily and looks fine to you, but she does indeed have a firm bump. You review her delivery records and find it was a difficult mid forceps one and that A. J. was described as having swelling over the left parietal region. Another cephalhematoma seems quite likely. You suggest watching the lump, but the parents are past reasoning and so you order AP and lateral skull films. What do you see?

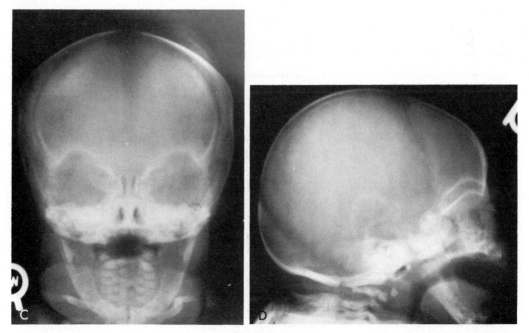

Figure 2–1c, d

There is soft tissue swelling over the left parietal bone seen most easily on the AP view. A fine rim of calcification is also seen over the swelling. The calcification is harder to detect on the lateral film but can be seen almost paralleling the upper margin of the parietal bone.

You show the film to A. J.'s parents and try to convince them that the lump will disappear slowly over the next several months. They are reluctant to believe you but at least agree to do nothing more at present. The mass follows your predictions and is no longer detectable at your nine month examination of A. J.

After a long labor, B. W. is finally delivered with forceps. You are asked to see the child because of a swollen, boggy head. Fearing skull trauma during the long delivery you order skull films. What are your findings?

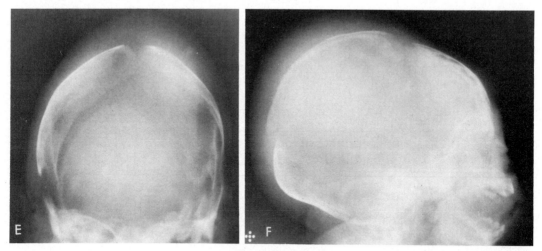

Figure 2–1e, f

There is a rather diffuse soft tissue swelling over the parietal and occipital regions that is not limited by the margins of a bone, unlike a cephalhematoma. The sutural overlapping is normal in the neonate and is due to "molding" during birth. The diffuse soft tissue swelling in this case is a caput succedaneum and is diffuse edema caused by birth trauma. No specific therapy is needed even though the appearance, as in B. W., can be quite alarming.

Cephalhematomas are well-known sequelae of childbirth. They are often associated with difficult labor and the use of forceps. They may occur with or without a skull fracture. The distinguishing feature of these hematomas is their limitation by the periosteum to a single bone, while the caput succedaneum is more diffuse in nature. Subgaleal hematomas can occur at any age and generally are caused by a specific injury. They are not confined to a single calvarial bone but are quite tense because they are confined by the galea aponeurotica, unlike the diffuse, fluctuant caput succedaneum. Cephalhematomas frequently develop a calcific rim within a few days of birth as in A. J. They usually resorb spontaneously over the first year of life but may also ossify and be slowly incorporated into the calvarium.

M. E., C. J., A. M., MR. P. C., MR. J. A., MRS. L. A. AND R. W.

Linear skull fractures would seem to be out of place in a book devoted to soft tissue trauma, but the presence of a linear fracture may serve as an indicator of significant trauma to the head; and associated soft tissue injury to the brain, including concussion or contusion, hemorrhage, epidural and subdural hematomas, can often be found. In addition, there are delayed complications of linear skull fractures of some clinical importance. While skull series are much less frequently performed now for suspected linear fracture than in the past, it may be important to determine that trauma has been the cause of an abnormality in the brain seen on CT. Trying to prove that a child has been battered or that an unconscious older person has suffered an injury rather than a spontaneous bleed will serve as examples.

Depressed skull fractures are an entirely different story. The bony fragments frequently cause brain damage and usually must be elevated. Bony fragments must be located carefully and the amount of depression rather precisely defined. CT can do this well, though appropriately positioned skull films can accomplish the same thing.

This case includes a spectrum of skull fractures and their associated soft tissue trauma. If the diagnostic approach to these cases seems repetitious, it is because this particular type of injury has few options in diagnosis.

M. E. was up on an old stepladder hanging the bunting for his 35th class reunion when he stretched a bit too far, lost his balance and crashed to the floor, bringing the stepladder down with him. The reunion committee rushed to his aid, but finding him unconscious, called an ambulance. He regained consciousness before the ambulance arrived but seemed quite confused. He is still disoriented when you see him in the emergency room. The emergency room physicians had already examined him, finding nothing wrong except swelling over the right side of his head and several other abrasions and bruises. They had ordered skull films, which you now review.

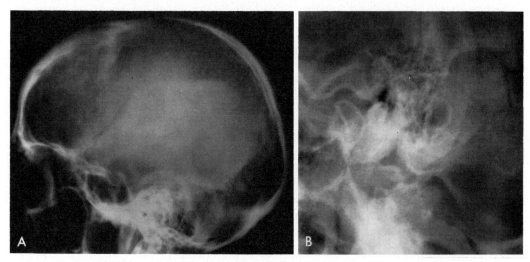

Figure 2–2a, b

There is a vertically oriented linear fracture of the right temporal bone which extends into the right mastoid air cells. You probably would not have ordered the skull films, but the presence of a fracture does mean that M. E. hit his head with some force. You are concerned about his continued confusion and request a CT scan to look for more serious problems. What abnormalities do you have in mind? What do you see on the sections illustrated? Remember, a CT scan of the head is viewed as if the reader were looking down on it from above, with the right side on the right and the left side on the left. This is different from a body CT scan, which is viewed in a mirror image, as is a plain film radiograph.

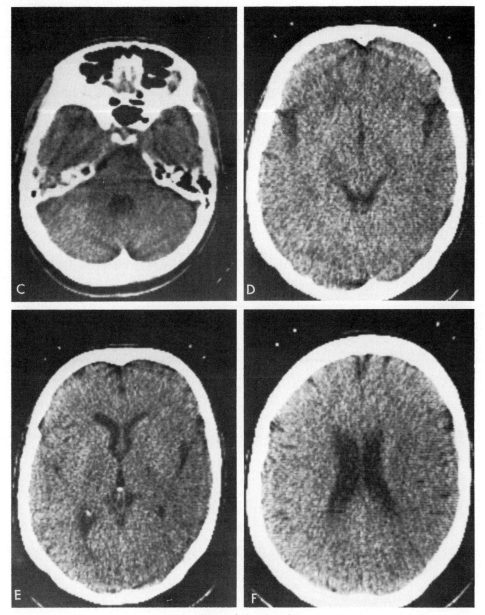

Figure 2–2c, d, e, f

You are concerned primarily about brain contusion or focal hemorrhage, though either a subdural or an epidural hematoma could be present. You are relieved to find the CT scan normal. The ventricles are symmetrical, and midline structures are midline. No areas of parenchymal or extra-axial hemorrhage are seen. These would be seen as areas of increased attenuation. The sulci are also symmetrical. While brain contusion has probably occurred in M. E., the injury is too subtle for CT to resolve. You admit M. E. for observation but tell him that he can probably plan on attending his reunion in two days, which he does do.

The circus had just been to town, inspiring C. J. to become a tight-rope walker. He tried a few fences and found them easy to balance on. Thus encouraged, he fastened a sturdy cable from his father's electrical shop between his porch railing and the house next door. He had no way to tighten the cable and it sagged markedly as he began to walk across it, making him lose his balance. He was only about seven feet above the driveway when he fell, but he hit the right side of his head very hard on the pavement and was momentarily unconscious. His audience of children helped him into the house, since he felt groggy and weak. When his mother heard the story and saw the swelling on the right side of his head, she insisted that C. J. go to see you.

C. J. has little of his usual teenage bravado showing when you see him. He has an extensive swelling over his right parietal area but complains of a left-sided headache. As you examine him for any neurologic deficits you think he is becoming increasingly confused so you order a CT scan to look for either extra-axial or intracerebral bleeding. Two sections are illustrated. What do you see, and are you surprised?

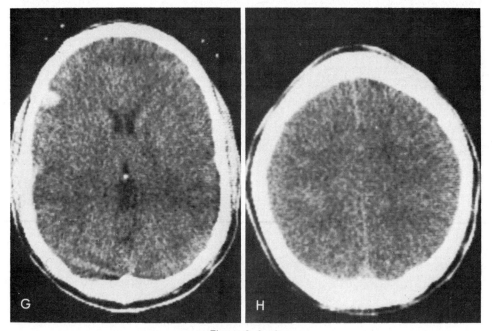

Figure 2–2g, h

Both sections show two small areas of increased attenuation in the left parietal lobe peripherally. These are focal areas of hemorrhage. No subdural hematoma is present, and no bleeding or contusion is seen on the right. The radiologist manipulates the bone window on the scanner but cannot demonstrate a fracture. While you are sure there is no depressed fracture, you wonder if there is a linear fracture on the right, so the radiologist obtains a right lateral and a PA view of the skull. What do you see?

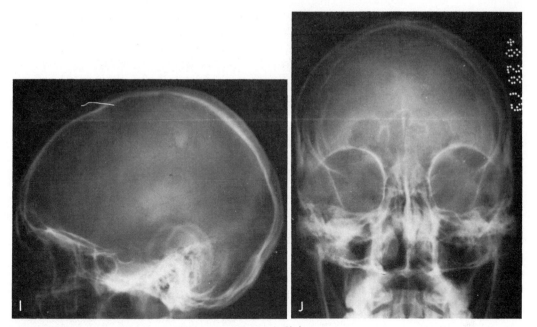

Figure 2–2i, j

There is a typical linear fracture which has a horizontal orientation located in the right parietal bone, possibly extending into the temporal bone. Do you see the fracture on the postero-anterior view? It is rather subtle but can be seen as two linear defects in the skull at about its broadest point. The fracture is markedly foreshortened by this projection. No fracture is seen on the left. Can you explain the CT observations in light of the skull films?

You might wonder if one of the studies is mislabelled. Both are correctly marked. The findings are those of a *contre-coup* injury. The brain can move to a limited degree in the skull. When the head is struck with sufficient force, the brain strikes the calvarium opposite the blow, causing brain injury which can be just a simple contusion but may also be more serious such as the hemorrhage in C. J. The fracture itself is rather insignificant and does not cross a major meningeal vascular groove, so there is not much risk of an epidural hematoma. There is, however, real damage to the brain.

C. J. is admitted for observation and, aside from his headache and soft tissue swelling, has no problems. Repeat limited CT scan five days later shows the blood to be resorbing and he is discharged. Delayed complications such as subdural hematomas are unlikely in C. J. and, in fact, none occur. Serious sequelae, such as seizures or chronic headaches, may be seen after contusion to the brain but young C. J., like most people with such injuries, is lucky. You see his mother a few months later and learn that C. J. has gone to join the circus school in Florida. She thinks he will probably become a juggler or a clown, since he has developed a dislike of heights.

At 13 months of age, A. M. has had more than his share of injuries. His parents, though loving, lack common sense, and A. M. is an inquisitive baby who began climbing up things weeks before he could stand. Earlier today he pulled himself up onto the railing at the top of the back door steps and promptly fell about six feet into the garden. He hit his head on a stake; his sister said it sounded like an egg breaking. Though he screamed as he fell, almost immediately after hitting the ground he became unresponsive. He had a small scalp laceration that bled a great deal and rapidly developed swelling on the left side of his head. Even A. M.'s parents were concerned by this series of events, so they bundled all the children into the car and have come to the emergency room.

When you see A. M., he is unresponsive and certainly has an impressive swelling of his head. You feel in the laceration and are quite sure there is a depressed skull fracture. You order skull films to confirm this impression. Two are shown. What do you see?

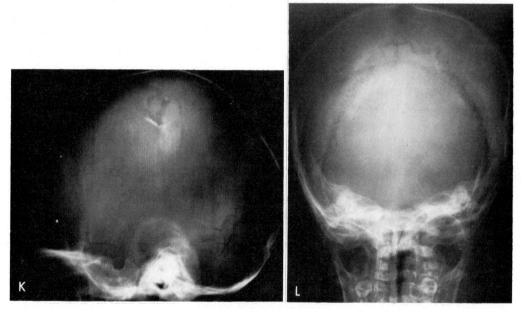

Figure 2–2k, l

The lateral film has the typical radiographic findings of a depressed skull fracture with regions of increased and decreased density caused by the overlapping of bony fragments and the fracture lines themselves. The degree of depression cannot be assessed on this film. The Towne view (Fig. 2–2l) is more help in assessing the amount of depression. At least one fragment is displaced well into the brain. The technologist suggests views tangential to the fracture to better demonstrate the depression. You concur and in a few minutes he returns with another film. What do you see now?

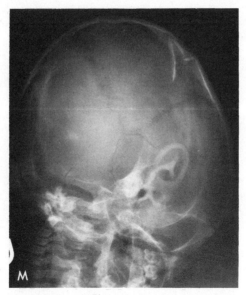

Figure 2–2m

This film demonstrates three depressed fragments all of which will need surgical elevation. You call a neurosurgeon who asks you to get a CT scan to evaluate brain injury while he drives to the hospital. You arrange for an emergency CT scan and watch the procedure. Three sections are illustrated. What are your thoughts?

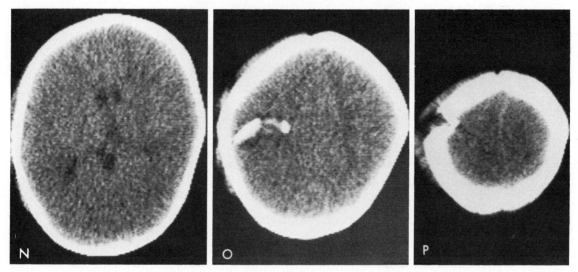

Figure 2–2n, o, p

The lowest section shows shift of midline structures to the right, but no subdural hematoma or parenchymal bleeding is seen. Soft tissue swelling of the scalp is present on the left and is more marked on the two higher sections, which also show the depressed fracture fragments and some surrounding edema but, amazingly, no bleeding. The last two sections are then displayed to better demonstrate the bone fragments.

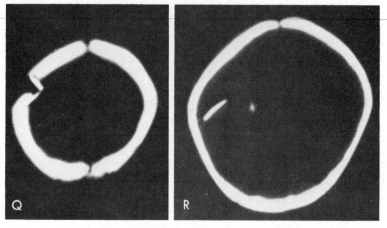

Figure 2–2q, r

The higher cut shows two bony fragments angling into the brain at the fracture itself. The lower section, below the fracture, shows two more fragments deep in brain substance. While you are looking at these bone window displays, the neurosurgeon arrives. He requests a measurement of the depth of the innermost fragment.

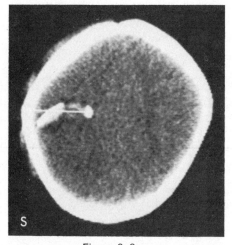

Figure 2–2s

The CT scanner can accurately provide direct measurements of this nature. In A. M. the deepest fragment was 43 mm deep to the inner table of the skull.

The depressed fragments are removed at surgery. The neurosurgeon says there is rather extensive brain damage in the path of the fragments. A. M. does not respond well at first, but when you see him a couple of weeks later, only the large dressing on his head is left to tell of his recent injury.

A. M. tolerated a rather major depressed skull fracture quite well. Mr. P. C. was not as lucky. He was pistol whipped by his grandson after refusing to give the boy the car. He was unresponsive when he was brought to the hospital. Skull films were obtained. What do you see on the two views illustrated?

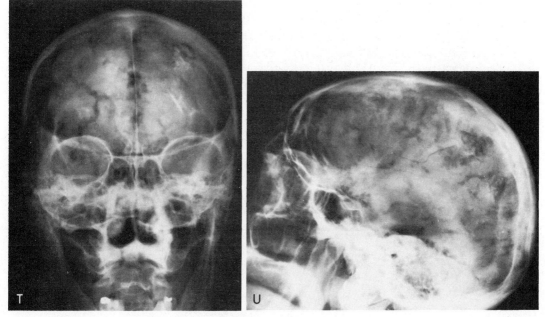

Figure 2–2t, u

Two depressed fractures are in evidence on each view. On the anteroposterior view, they are seen on the left and appear primarily as areas of increased bony density. On the lateral, the two fractures are located posteriorly in the parietal bone. More striking, and somewhat confusing, is air over the surface of the brain. The air must come from a fracture that communicates with an airspace such as the mastoid air cells, tympanic cavity, or any of the paranasal sinuses or even the nasal cavity itself. Pneumocephalus is of no clinical significance except that it should alert the radiologist and the doctors caring for the patient that such a fracture has occurred.

Mr. P. C. is sent for a CT scan, which shows several areas of cerebral hemorrhage in addition to defining the depth of the bony fragments. Despite efforts to improve his status, he dies about six hours after arrival at the hospital.

Depressed skull fractures are almost invariably accompanied by significant brain injury. Evaluation of the nature and extent of the soft tissue injury is useful to the clinician both in planning therapy and in determining patient prognosis.

Mr. J. A. was robbed by three teenagers one night, and when he attempted to resist the hoodlums, he was pushed violently to the ground and kicked several times on the head. His wife sent for an ambulance and called you. When you meet the A.'s in the emergency room you are struck by how confused Mr. J. A. is. He also has two cuts that are still bleeding. One is over his left eyebrow and the other, a larger one, is at the back of his head on the right.

Mr. J. A. is injured severely enough that you decide to order a CT scan to demonstrate any significant intracranial trauma, but before he goes to CT, you suture his lacerations. The one over the left eyebrow is quite superficial and is easily closed; the other laceration is irregular, quite long and extends to the skull. Before suturing this one you obtain a limited skull series to rule out a depressed skull fracture. What do you see on the PA and right lateral skull films illustrated here?

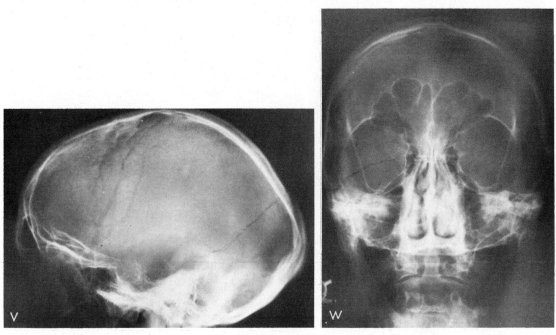

Figure 2–2v, w

There is a linear skull fracture on the right that extends from almost the midline through the parietal bone well into the temporal bone. It may even extend into the base of the skull. There is no evidence of depression of the fracture fragments. You may have noticed an ovoid region of increased density on the lateral film located in the parietal region. This is dirt, matted in the blood in his hair.

You clean the wound, suture it and send Mr. J. A. for his CT scan. He seems less confused than when you first saw him, but he remains belligerent and uncooperative. You are not surprised when the radiologist says that the scans were done with the shortest possible scanning time and are still limited by patient motion. Two sections are illustrated. What is your opinion?

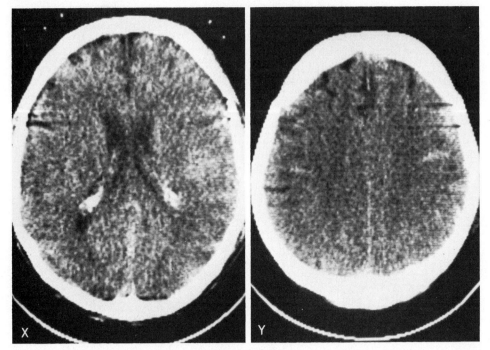

Figure 2-2x, y

The first section is at the level of the lateral ventricles, which are normal in size and position. Lateral to the right lateral ventricle is a poorly defined rounded area of increased attenuation. No sulci are seen in this region. There are additional vague streaky areas of increased attenuation adjacent to the calvarium. The second section demonstrates sulci on the left, but none are seen on the right and once again patchy areas of increased density are present. These findings are those of brain contusion with some petecchial hemorrhage and edema. No large hematoma is present, and no subdural or epidural hematoma is present.

Mr. J. A. is admitted for observation primarily because of his confusion. Within a day, he is nearly back to normal mentally, though he has some rather incredible ecchymoses. When Mr. J. A. becomes impatient to go home, you discharge him with instructions to come to your office to have his stitches removed. On that day, he seems fine and you think that the entire episode has passed rather well.

About six weeks later, Mr. J. A.'s son calls. He had come to visit his parents at his mother's urgent request. She felt that J. A. had gone downhill rapidly after the stitches were removed, and his son finds him very much changed. Worried, you arrange to meet them at the emergency room. When you see Mr. J. A., you are horrified. He is gaunt and unkempt, his speech is incoherent and his attention span is very limited. Physical examination adds little except for bilateral positive Babinski's, diffuse hyperreflexia and a suggestion of papilledema. You decide to get another CT scan, though you have little idea what is going on. Two sections at levels similar to those you have already seen are demonstrated on the following page. What do you see?

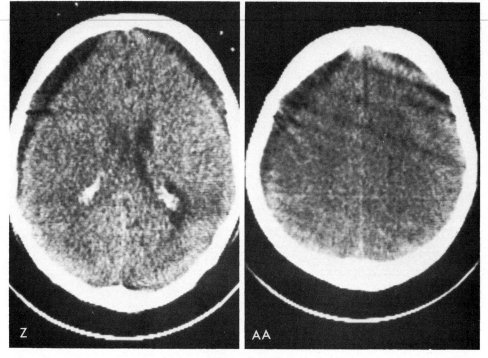

Figure 2–2z, aa

There are bilateral crescentic areas of low attenuation between the brain and the calvarium. This is the typical appearance of a subacute or chronic subdural hematoma. Contrast material has not been given, so you cannot look for enhancement in the membrane. The subdural collections are a delayed complication of the original head injury. Venous tears occur at the time of the original trauma, but acute brain swelling compresses the veins, impeding formation of a subdural hematoma. Bleeding then occurs when the swelling diminishes.

Mr. J. A. has deteriorated markedly over the last six weeks and you wonder what approach will be best for him. Both the neurologic and neurosurgical consultants recommend aspiration, which proceeds uneventfully. However, Mr. J. A. does not improve significantly after drainage and dies three days later.

Mrs. L. A., a 43 year old female, is sent in for an insurance physical. She denies any illness, and your routine physical examination is unremarkable. You are about through with her physical examination when you notice a swelling on the back of her head. Palpation reveals a somewhat tense, but also pulsatile mass in the right posterior parietal region. When questioned about this, she says it has been there for many years but she hasn't mentioned it for fear of increasing her insurance rate. You decide to get skull films. What do you make of the hole in the head?

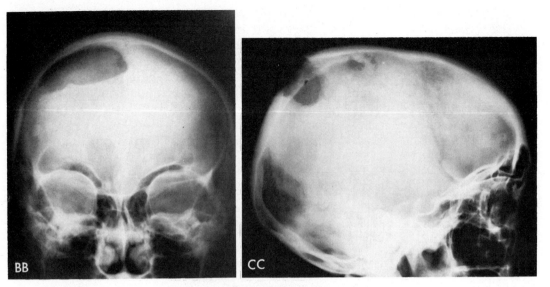

Figure 2–2bb, cc

Initially, you are alarmed by the large area of bony destruction. Close inspection with the consulting radiologist is reassuring, however. The margins of the lesions are sharp, and when seen in tangent, the outer table is beveled and elevated. These are findings of a slow-growing lesion that is expanding from within outward. The lesion is characteristic of a "growing fracture" or post-traumatic leptomeningeal cyst.

R. W. is a young girl whose misfortune it was to be hit by a drunk driver while she was riding her bicycle to school one morning. She suffered many injuries, including a ruptured spleen and shattered right femur. You were called to see her because of a skull fracture of the left frontal region and bilateral subdural hematomas. The fracture was extensive and rather stellate, crossing midline to involve the right orbital roof. You treated the right subdural by drainage through burr holes, but the left one required a large flap to clear.

R. W. has a stormy few days but is clearly on the mend five days after admission when she begins to complain of a runny nose. You immediately start worrying about leakage of cerebrospinal fluid, and your impression is confirmed by the presence of glucose in the fluid. You review the admission skull series and the CT scan and request repeat lateral and anteroposterior skull films. None show a fracture involving any of the sinuses or base of the skull, but there is no doubt that the left frontal fracture could extend into the cribriform plate. You feel it is important to know where the cerebrospinal fluid leakage is occurring, since surgical repair may become necessary. You can choose among several diagnostic tests. A radioactive tracer can be injected into the lumbar subarachnoid space and scans obtained to look for the leaking focus. The isotopic procedure, though very useful in locating a leak, does not give detailed anatomic information. Placement of pledgets in selected locations which are then reviewed for accumulated radioactivity, with the highest activity indicating the approximate site of leakage, can help. You could do close interval high resolution CT scans of the cribriform plate for multiplanar reconstruction. CT is often performed before and after injection of water soluble contrast into the subarachnoid space in an attempt to see actual leakage. In this case, however, you decide to start with conventional tomography.

What do you see on the lateral tomographic cut that is illustrated here?

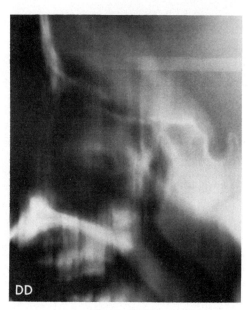

Figure 2–2dd

There is clearly a fracture of the cribriform plate with some slight depression of the ventral fracture fragments. Communication with ethmoid air cells explains, in part, the runny nose R. W. is experiencing.

It is necessary to repair the dural tear, but R. W. does very well after surgery. She has to go to summer session to make up for all the school days she missed, but by fall she is once again riding her bicycle to class.

MS. A. B. AND MASTER O. H.

When the ambulance crew phones ahead that they are bringing in a young woman with a head injury who is rapidly losing consciousness, you alert the CT technician and meet Ms. A. B. as she is wheeled into the emergency department. Her boyfriend says she was painting a large wall mural when she lost her balance and fell about fifteen feet. Her fall had been largely cushioned by a lilac bush, but she hit her head on a rock and was out cold for a few minutes. On regaining consciousness, she tried to stand, felt very dizzy and collapsed. An ambulance was called and when it arrived, A. B. was able to tell the driver what hospital she wanted to go to, but a minute or two later the ambulance attendant could get no verbal response from her. That was when they phoned you.

Ms. A. B. does respond to pain, but nothing else. A quick examination is of little help except she does have swelling above both ears, which is perhaps slightly more prominent on the right where she hit the rock. The swelling on the left side is a bit of a puzzle, but you don't worry about it. Vital signs are stable so you go ahead with the CT head scan. Four sections done without intravenous contrast material are shown. What is your opinion?

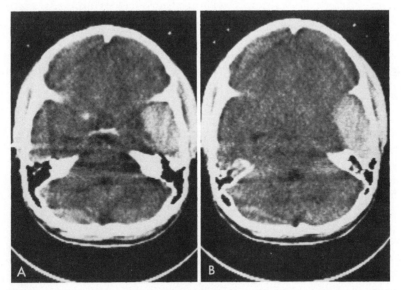

Figure 2–3a, b

The first section shows bilateral subgaleal hematomas, but much more striking is the large area of high attenuation in the right temporal region. This area of bleeding lies outside the brain substance and is displacing the brain from the cranial vault. The suprasellar cistern is compressed, suggesting impending uncal herniation. The second scan 1 cm cephalad again shows the rather well-defined biconvex area of bleeding and the subgaleal hematomas.

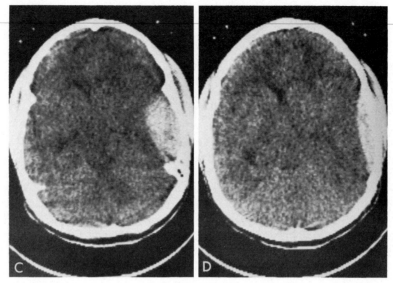

Figure 2–3c, d

The third section demonstrates the mass effect with displacement of the lateral ventricles across the midline to the left. The right lateral ventricle is effaced. The final section again shows mass effect and shift of the ventricles. The bleed is smaller at this level but maintains its well-defined biconvex configuration.

The neurosurgeon arrives in the CT control room just as the examination is started. He concurs with a diagnosis of epidural hematoma made by the radiologist and arranges for immediate drainage, which occurs about two hours after the injury.

A. B. responds well to evacuation of the epidural hematoma. She cannot really remember the events that surrounded her hospitalization, but she is soon well enough for discharge.

No explanation is ever found for her left subgaleal hematoma. She goes back to her mural painting, and several weeks later when you attend dedication ceremonies you recognize the neurosurgeon and yourself among the faces portrayed.

The quick and easy diagnosis of an epidural hematoma in Ms. A. B. makes you reflect on the many advantages of practicing medicine in the era of computed tomography. Then you remember that only six weeks earlier you had another patient with an epidural hematoma when the CT scanner was "down." That meant that O. H., a sweet six month old boy, had to have an emergency cerebral angiogram under general anesthesia to make the diagnosis. All had gone smoothly, even the percutaneous catheterization of the small femoral artery, but it was nearly three hours before the study was complete, including set-up time and anesthesia. Still, the outcome was good and O. H. went home in a few days after surgery. The angiographic examination requires skill to perform and interpret. Have a look at these interesting arterial phase films.

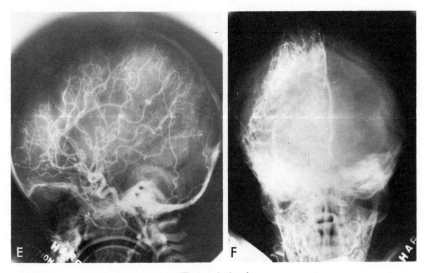

Figure 2–3e, f

The lateral arterial phase film is not dramatic, though to a trained eye it is certainly abnormal. The findings on the AP projection are striking. There is a large biconcave avascular space separating the vessels of the brain from the calvarium. These are the classic findings of an extracerebral hematoma. The lenticular shape is characteristic of an acute epidural hematoma, as is the medial displacement of the middle meningeal artery. Look at the repeat figure with arrows on the middle meningeal artery.

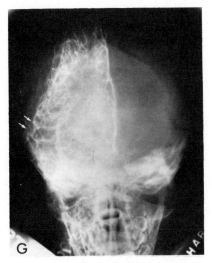

Figure 2–3g

Since the middle meningeal artery runs in the dura, the hematoma must be between the dura and the calvarium, confirming the presence of an epidural hematoma.

Angiography continues to have a role in head trauma, but the indications are now much narrower. Angiography is needed to evaluate most vascular complications of head injury such as traumatic aneurysms, arteriovenous fistulae or vascular occlusions. For routine head trauma, CT will usually be speedy, simple and completely diagnostic. Epidural hematomas can expand quickly and compress the brain, causing brain damage and death, so rapid diagnosis is very important.

K. D., D. L., J. G., H. R. AND D. D.

In contrast to the epidural hematomas discussed in Case 2–3, where speed in diagnosis and therapy is frequently critical in saving the patient, subdural hematomas generally have a somewhat slower evolution. Even so, the workup of subdural hematomas should be pursued with reasonable speed, since they can cause serious compression of the brain.

Before the introduction of CT scanning, subdural hematomas were evaluated by isotopic scanning and by selective carotid angiography. While isotopic scanning is rarely used now, very thin subdural hematomas can be missed at CT, and therefore angiography may occasionally be needed.

Mr. D. heard K. D. come in. She was awfully noisy and clumsy, and he thought he would speak to her in the morning about being more considerate. He opened an eye to see what the time was and was annoyed to see it was after 3:00 A.M. Just then, his daughter made a great racket and he jumped out of bed to investigate. K. D. was crumpled at the foot of the stairs, smelling of liquor and vomit. She would not get up, so he went angrily back to bed. Being jilted by a fiancé two weeks before the wedding is no reason to stay out late and get stinking drunk, he thought.

He overslept in the morning and was horrified to see his daughter, just as he had left her, at the foot of the stairs. He could not arouse her and, highly concerned, called an ambulance. You meet the ambulance when it arrives at the emergency room. K. D. does look awful. She has bruises over her face and a left parietal scalp laceration that has bled copiously over her clothes. Further examination reveals bruises on her body and legs. She is responsive to pain and to insistent commands, but will not talk to you. Her right side seems weak and her pupils are unequal. You order an emergency CT head scan and try to reassure Mr. D., who is feeling terribly guilty and is worrying his daughter will die.

Four sections from the CT scan are shown on the following page. When you see the first scan illustrated come up on the video monitor, you call a neurosurgeon. Why? What else do you see on the higher sections?

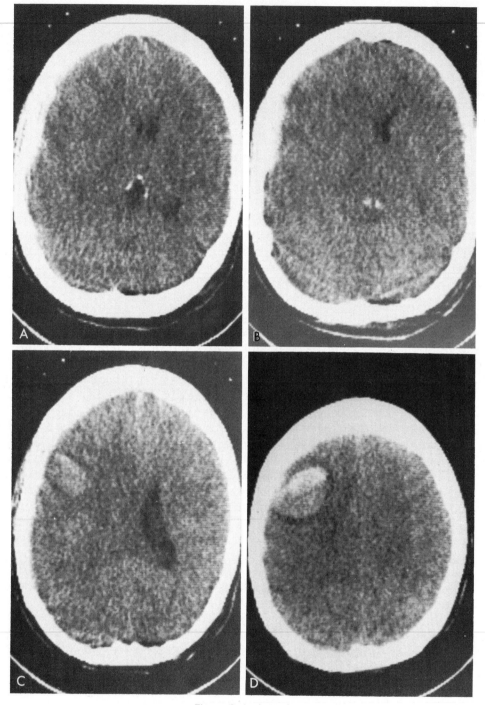

Figure 2–4a, b, c, d

The first section shows marked shift of the lateral ventricles to the right. The left hemisphere occupies considerably more space than the right, indicating swelling. In addition, there is an acute subdural hematoma on the left that is seen as a high attenuation, almost linear density along the inner margin of the skull. A subgaleal hematoma lies under the laceration.

The second section is 1 cm higher. The shift, the edema and the subdural hematoma are all seen again. The degree of swelling seems out of proportion to the subdural hematoma, so you are not particularly surprised by the new finding on the third section, 2 cm cephalad. There is an intracerebral hemorrhage in the left frontoparietal region seen on this section and on the final cut 1 cm higher. The zone of edema is more sharply defined on these cuts.

K. D. is placed on steroids to reduce the swelling. She responds rather well for about 36 hours but then begins to deteriorate, so both the subdural and intracerebral hematomas are evacuated. Aside from an aspiration pneumonia, she does very well and has little discernible neurologic deficit when she leaves the hospital.

⚜

You are called to the emergency ward to see D. L., who has been found wandering about in the central business district of town. He does not know his name, but a search of his wallet reveals that he is a well-known businessman. A call to his home is alarming. His wife has not seen him for three days and has reported him missing to the police.

A physical examination reveals unequal pupils, brisk reflexes and an upgoing great toe on the left. There is a prominent bruise on the right temporoparietal region and other minor cuts and abrasions. The patient's orientation and level of consciousness are steadily worsening as you observe him. Intracranial trauma is clearly on your mind, and you order a "stat" CT scan and call in a neurosurgeon.

The radiologist calls and tells you to come over to the scanner. You are joined by the neurosurgeon, who calls the operating room after a glance at the scan. What do you see on the non-contrast sections shown on the following page?

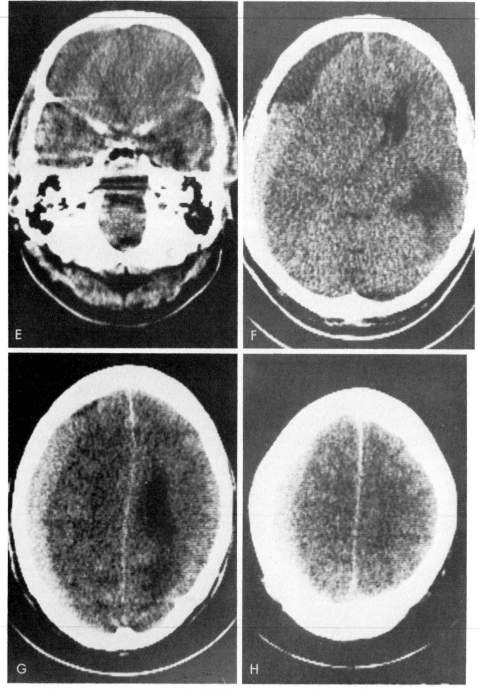

Figure 2–4e, f, g, h

There is a large, crescentic collection that displaces the right hemisphere from the calvarium. The midline structures are shifted to the left, and the right lateral ventricle is collapsed while the left lateral is enlarged. This is indicative of 'trapping' of the left lateral ventricle secondary to the subfalcine herniation of brain, with resulting obstruction of the foramen of Monro and subsequent dilatation of the ventricle because of continued CSF elaboration by the choroid plexus.

Careful inspection of the crescentic collection shows that it has two components; one of these is of higher attenuation than brain and is dependent in its distribution. A rather straight line separates this component from the anterior, low attenuating component. Section 2–4f illustrates this finding best. In the uppermost section only the higher attenuation component is seen.

This is a classical appearance for a subacute subdural hematoma. The crescentic configuration results from the tendency of subdural bleeding to spread diffusely over the brain from its point of origin. The two components are the result of separation of the hematoma into high attenuation clots and "supernatant" plasma.

These findings are confirmed at surgery, and D. L. recovers rapidly. He is reluctant to discuss his trauma and lost three days and soon checks out of the hospital.

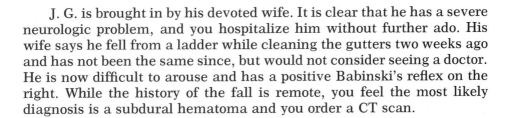

J. G. is brought in by his devoted wife. It is clear that he has a severe neurologic problem, and you hospitalize him without further ado. His wife says he fell from a ladder while cleaning the gutters two weeks ago and has not been the same since, but would not consider seeing a doctor. He is now difficult to arouse and has a positive Babinski's reflex on the right. While the history of the fall is remote, you feel the most likely diagnosis is a subdural hematoma and you order a CT scan.

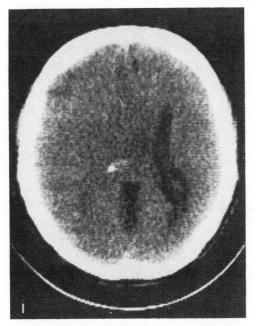

Figure 2–4i

Only a single section is illustrated. The findings, while quite dramatic, could be missed by an inexperienced observer. The left lateral ventricle is completely effaced and is displaced to the right. The focal white density is calcified choroid plexus of the left lateral ventricle, which identifies its location. There is, therefore, a marked mass effect on the left side of the brain, but it is difficult to determine the cause. These findings are those of an "isodense" subdural hematoma.

During the evolution of a subdural hematoma from acute to chronic the extra-axial blood collection will pass through a phase when the contents are virtually identical to brain in their ability to attenuate x-rays. Because of this, the collection is not seen as separate from the adjacent brain on the CT scan. In some patients the collection may have small areas of higher or lower attenuation that help to identify it, as is actually true of this case. In other cases only secondary signs such as mass effect or the presence of peripheral contrast enhancement can be used to identify the abnormality. This can be especially difficult if the subdural collections are bilateral and symmetrical so that the mass effects balance one another.

J. G. does quite well after the evacuation of his large subdural hematoma, but his memory of the last two weeks is poor and he is very angry with you because of the large bandage on his head.

H. R. is also brought in by his wife, who is concerned about his changing behavior. As he has gotten older, he has become a binge drinker and is often irritable. Now he is complaining of headaches, is lethargic and has an unsteady gait.

Your physical examination reveals him to be more disheveled than in the recent past. His gait is ataxic, and he has brisk deep tendon reflexes only on the right. He complains repeatedly of a headache and wants to go home. He denies any injury but does have a nearly healed cut on the right side of his head. His wife says this happened about a month ago during a drinking bout.

You order a CT scan, suspecting trauma, though an intracerebral mass of any type could have the same presentation. The sections illustrated were obtained before the administration of intravenous contrast material. What do they show?

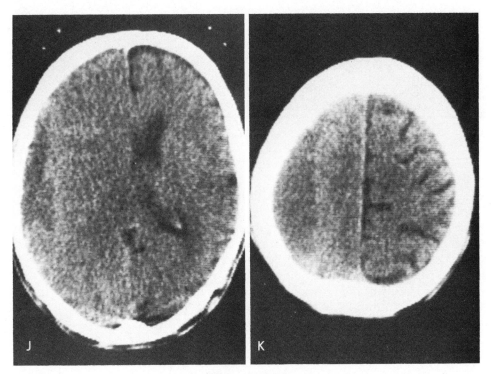

Figure 2-4j, k

The lower section is at the level of the lateral ventricles. There is a marked shift of the ventricular and midline structures to the right, with effacement of the left lateral ventricle. There is an irregular area of decreased attenuation peripherally. In the more cephalic section the area of decreased attenuation has a more crescentic configuration, though posteriorly it bulges inward. The cortical sulci are obliterated on the left. The findings are those of a chronic subdural hematoma, and the radiologist has given intravenous contrast material to H. R. to demonstrate any membrane. What do you see on sections done at the same levels as the first two but after the contrast material (following page)?

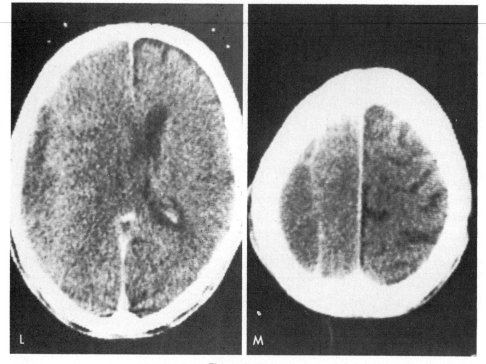

Figure 2–4l, m

The contrast material has enhanced the membrane. This is most easily seen on the higher section.

The CT findings in H. R. are characteristic of a chronic subdural hematoma. As the collection of blood breaks down, it draws in fluid. While collection may be quite proteinaceous it attenuates x-rays less than normal brain. The linear area of contrast enhancement seen at the inner margin of the collection is due to a vascular inflammatory membrane about the subdural hematoma which becomes stained by the contrast material. Such membranes may actually calcify in very long-standing hematomas.

H. R. is taken to the operating room that night. A large subdural collection, containing 75 cc of material that looks like crankcase oil, is found on the left.

As we have seen, extracerebral hematomas have a variety of appearances depending on their location and duration. In the acute state, the hematoma is generally more dense than brain, though it should be noted that in very anemic patients, acute hematomas may be isodense. Epidural hematomas tend to be lenticular in shape when acute and subdural hematomas tend to be crescentic. As subdural hematomas evolve they become less dense, and they become less crescentic as they imbibe fluid. Chronic subdural hematomas also develop adjacent inflammatory membranes, which can be identified by contrast medium infusion.

D. D. is returning from a ski trip when he skids on an icy mountain road, demolishing his car against some trees. He is found dazed and wandering by the road by passing motorists who bring him to the emergency room. He has a nasty gash on his left temple and is disoriented, but there are no focal neurologic signs. Skull films show a linear fracture of the left parietal bone. His laceration is sutured and you order a CT brain scan. What do you see on his examination done after contrast infusion?

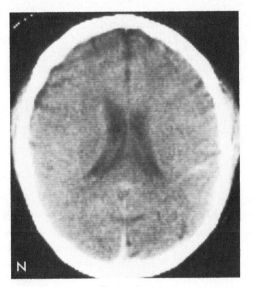

Figure 2–4n

There is a scalp hematoma on the left. The left lateral ventricle and cortical sulci are somewhat effaced. These findings are compatible with brain swelling caused by a contusion. There is also a small high attenuation focus in the left cortex, perhaps a small area of hemorrhage. Since no large intracerebral or extracerebral hematoma is seen, you relax and admit D. D. for observation.

D. D. continues to complain of headache and becomes quite abusive and demanding over the next three days, so you decide to order a repeat CT scan partly to satisfy him and partly to look for delayed bleeding. You are surprised when the radiologist calls you down to see the scan on the following page. What now?

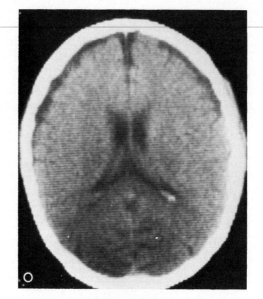

Figure 2–4o

The contusion is resolving, but there are now bilateral crescentic low attenuation areas in both frontal regions. These look like small chronic subdural hematomas, but you know that there was no subdural collection three days ago and so these collections must be subdural hygromas. These are more common in children than in adults and are usually caused by an arachnoid tear which allows subarachnoid fluid to enter the potential subdural space. They may become chronic and require tapping or may resolve spontaneously.

D. D. is pleased that there is something to account for his complaints and feels quite smug. The subdural hygromas resolve over the next few weeks, and you and the nursing staff are pleased to see the last of him.

As you have read, linear skull fractures are, of themselves, of no clinical significance in contrast to the injury caused by depressed fractures. However, concomitant brain injury or laceration of dural or meningeal blood vessels may be serious. The presence of a linear skull fracture should alert the clinician to the possibility of significant associated trauma. D. D. illustrates both an unusual complication of a linear fracture and a differential diagnostic problem of hematoma versus hygroma.

MRS. B. B. AND MRS. C. B.

Depressed skull fractures, epidural hematomas and subdural hematomas are all rather specific abnormalities that can be well diagnosed and for which appropriate treatment can be planned. Intracerebral bleeding, brain contusion and concussion are sometimes easy to diagnose but can be difficult to define. Many such lesions will clear over time with supportive treatment, while some are life-threatening and require surgery. Before the development of CT scanning, such injuries were very difficult to diagnose, since angiography can demonstrate only a diffuse mass effect in both frank hemorrhage and brain contusion. Therapy was based on clinical observations. CT scanning gives a much more specific diagnosis with little risk to the patient. More important, the question of parenchymal injury can be answered in a very short time, facilitating appropriate therapy.

Mrs. B. B. and Mrs. C. B. illustrate some of the problems that can be encountered with actual brain injuries.

By all logic, Mrs. B. B. should have been moribund when she appeared in your office. As it was, both she and Mrs. C. B. had very similar histories and presentations. Both women had been victims of purse snatchers and both had fallen, striking their heads on the sidewalk. Both women had been helped by passersby, had made out police reports and had gone home.

Mrs. B. B., who was 76, called her daughter to tell her what had happened. She complained of headache and some unsteadiness, so that the daughter became concerned and went to her mother's home. Finding her mother rather shaken, she brings her to the emergency room where you meet them. Mrs. B. B. is more confused than usual and has papilledema and some questionable left-sided weakness. You wonder aloud if she has a concussion, and her daughter reminds you she is on long-term anticoagulation. You discuss the problem with a neurologist, who suggests a CT scan — the idea you were entertaining. Arrangements are made for this study and you also draw blood for a prothrombin time. The radiologist calls you when he views the first scan and he sounds somewhat excited. You understand his concern when you review the study. Four sections are illustrated on the following page. What are your observations and conclusions?

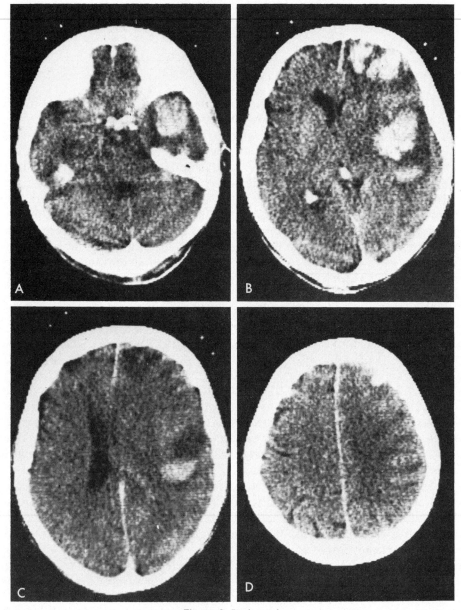

Figure 2–5a, b, c, d

Multiple areas of high attenuation are seen. All are areas of hemorrhage and are on the right. There is shift of midline structures to the left with effacement of the right lateral ventricle. There is some edema around the larger areas of hemorrhage. Sulci are effaced on the right but are still normal on the left.

Mrs. B. B. has obviously bled in several areas of her brain. What is surprising is how little the bleeding is affecting her. You admit Mrs. B. B., stop her coumadin for the time being and call in the neurologist to see her. Initially, she develops increased weakness and confusion, but then she improves and is transferred to a convalescent hospital after 16 days. One month after admission when you are about to send her home, you get a follow-up scan. One section is illustrated.

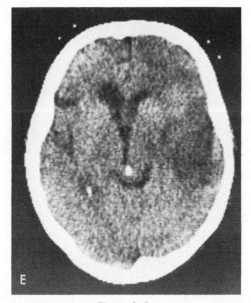

Figure 2–5e

The high attenuation area is gone, replaced by a large area of lower attenuation. The shift has also diminished. The decrease in attenuation is due to resorption of hemoglobin from the bleed, with some continuing edema.

All in all, Mrs. B. B. has done extremely well. In fact, you never understand why she was not much sicker. Perhaps she had enough cerebral atrophy to absorb the increased mass caused by bleeding with little compression of vital structures.

Mrs. C. B. is only 46. She has been your patient for some years and you know she is not a complainer nor does she magnify her symptoms. She calls late the evening of her mugging and says she has a severe frontal headache that is not responding to aspirin. With Mrs. B. B. fresh in your mind, you suggest that she take no more aspirin. She does not want any narcotics and says she will see you in the morning if the headache isn't better.

She is waiting for you when you reach your office the next day and says the headache is even worse. She has noticed no other problems, and your physical examination is not helpful. In view of her recent head trauma, you decide to get a CT scan. Three sections are illustrated on the following page. Do you see any abnormality?

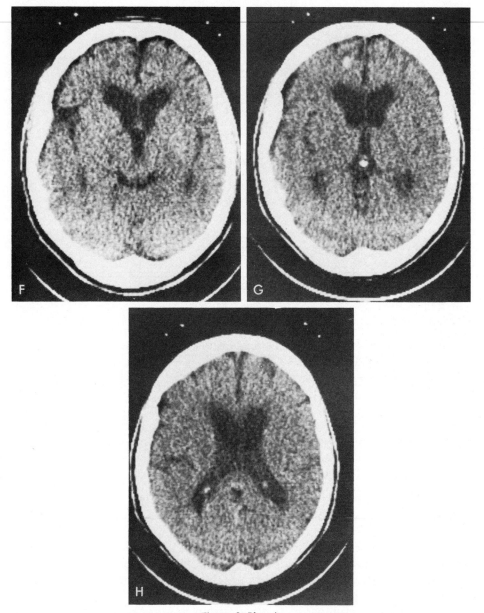

Figure 2–5f, g, h

Perhaps what surprises you most are the slightly prominent lateral and third ventricles along with big sulci and subarachnoid space. You would not have suspected atrophy in Mrs. C. B. More important, the middle section shows a rather discrete area of high attenuation. It is not as dense as the pineal calcification and has a ring of diminished attenuation around it. This is a small intracerebral bleed, and it is undoubtedly the source of her headache.

As a precautionary measure, you admit Mrs. C. B. to the hospital but, after a day, her headache is lessening and she is anxious to be about her business, so you discharge her. Limited follow-up CT scan two weeks later shows complete resorption of the blood with no residual abnormality.

Mrs. B. B. and Mrs. C. B. are graphic examples of the use of CT in providing a rapid and simple method for diagnosing intraparenchymal cerebral hemorrhage. Though a lumbar puncture will often indicate that there has been bleeding, it does not localize the site and is dangerous in patients with raised intracranial pressure. Cerebral angiography will demonstrate a mass but does not directly demonstrate the bleeding itself. CT is therefore the procedure of choice in patients in whom bleeding is suspected.

CASE 2–6:

MR. G. H.

Penetrating trauma to the brain almost invariably will require surgical intervention if the patient is to survive. The nature and timing of such surgery will depend on the injury, and any diagnostic maneuvers will be tailored to the needs of the specific patient. CT is a fine method for determining presence and location of foreign bodies, as well as the extent of brain injury. However, skull films and angiography will play a useful role in many patients. Skull films can be used to locate radiopaque foreign bodies and angiography can be used to look for injury to blood vessels, which will help determine prognosis as well as define what type of surgery must be undertaken.

In penetrating trauma, perhaps more than in any other type of injury in this chapter, diagnosis must be tailored to the precise dilemma rather than to a routine.

Mr. G. H. was walking through the park earlier this evening with two friends when they were suddenly surrounded by a group of ten or twelve children who pushed and shoved them, demanding money. Unable to believe the children could do any harm, they tried to break out of the pack only to have the largest girl brandish a gun. She fired it once to prove she could, and all three men handed over their wallets and started to run as the children squabbled over the contents. Sadly, the girl shot at them as they ran, hitting Mr. G. H. on the left side of the head. He fell, the children scattered into the park and one friend went to call an ambulance while the second stood guard.

The ambulance attendant calls you to the emergency room shortly after they pick up G. H., who is unconscious. He sees no exit wound, but there is an entrance wound posteriorly on the left. While waiting for the ambulance to arrive you arrange for an emergency CT scan to evaluate the extent of tissue damage and identify any hemorrhage either into the brain or around it. When G. H. arrives, you find that his right side is flaccid, that he responds only to deep pain but that his vital signs are stable, so you send him for the CT scan. What do you see on these non-contrast scans?

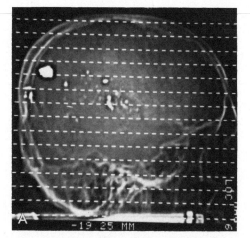

Figure 2–6a

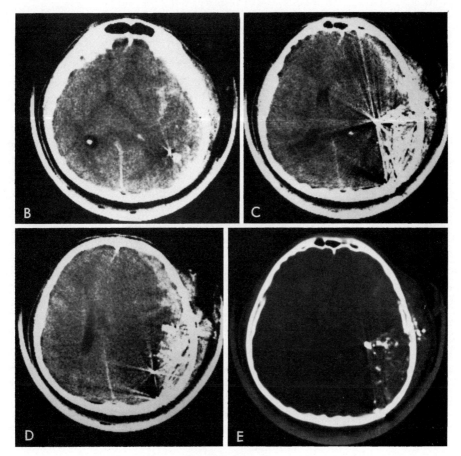

Figure 2–6b, c, d, e

The initial film is the preliminary view. The dotted lines indicate where the sections of the study have been made. You should notice that no angulation has been used, so the CT images will have an appearance slightly different from most of the others in this chapter. The many metallic fragments in the brain are readily identified. Some are quite large and have artifactual halos. Metallic objects this large will also degrade the actual CT images, but the four sections illustrated demonstrate that diagnostically useful information can be obtained even in the presence of serious artifacts. The first three CT scans are displayed for soft tissue and the fourth is a "bone window" display of the second section. The many metallic fragments are confined to the left posterior parietal area. There is a large accumulation of blood in the left subdural space and a marked shift to the right. You should have noticed the position of the lateral ventricles. Aside from the marked shift, there is effacement of most of the body of the left lateral ventricle. Cisterns and the third and fourth ventricles are not seen. While this could be due to the artifacts, it is more likely that the marked injury to the brain with secondary swelling is the cause. Herniation of the uncus and tonsils is a serious concern.

Mr. G. H. is started on high dose steroids and taken to surgery where much brain is debrided. Initially, the neurosurgeon is somewhat optimistic about the situation, but G. H. lapses into a deep coma and dies about ten hours after his injury.

CASE 2-7:

MR. V. B., R. B., B. S. AND A. A.

This group of patients all have suffered injury to the spinal cord. As with the brain, accurate, prompt diagnosis will diminish, if not reverse, the long-term effects of these injuries, so most should be treated as true emergencies.

Mr. V. B., an ardent dune buggy enthusiast, is brought to the emergency room after an accident in which he was thrown violently from his vehicle, smashing into a boulder. When he tried to get up, he found he could not move his right side. Friends carefully moved him onto the floor of a camper, but by the time you see him the paralysis has progressed to involve the left leg. Physical examination reveals that in fact there is anesthesia from the shoulders down. Your first thought is a cervical spine fracture. Carefully positioned AP and lateral films are unremarkable. Oblique views also are normal.

The consulting neurosurgeon thinks that the physical findings are those of cervical cord damage, possibly from an epidural spinal hematoma that could be relieved surgically. What test would you request?

A myelogram is the best way to separate a cord lesion from an extramedullary lesion and one is requested. What do you see?

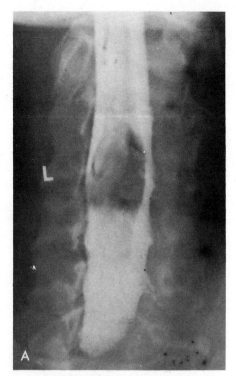

Figure 2-7a

A single view from the myelogram shows the cervical cord surround-ed by Pantopaque, an oily contrast medium. There is an area of fusiform enlargement of the cord extending over a length of two vertebral segments. The finding of a focal mass in the cord is present in all views and, in the context of trauma, is most likely caused by bleeding and swelling in the cord. Note that contrast medium flows around the enlarged cord and that there is no block in the spinal canal.

A conservative approach was elected for V. B., and his neurologic deficit does not progress. After several months he recovers some func-tion.

Contusion and hemorrhage into the cord may occur with or without fracture of the vertebra. The myelographic appearance of both is a localized enlargement of the cord. Not infrequently, the enlargement is great enough to cause a complete block. Current CT techniques do not resolve the cord with sufficient detail to be of use in this situation but undoubtedly will do so in the near future.

R. B., a day laborer who was injured on the job, is brought by his fellows for examination. It seems he became entangled with a winch which threw him forcefully. He complains of pain in the right side of the neck and arm. Cervical spine radiographs show a fracture of the dorsal arch and body of the sixth cervical vertebra.

A careful physical examination reveals right triceps weakness and diminished sensation in the right thumb. Because of the neurologic findings, a cervical myelogram is requested. A single oblique view is illustrated. What does it show?

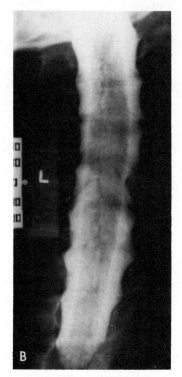

Figure 2–7b

There is a sharply marginated ovoid filling defect on the right adjacent to the sixth cervical vertebra that is interfering with filling of nerve root sleeve. While an extruded cervical disc could have a similar appearance, in the presence of trauma, a small extradural hematoma is more likely. This diagnosis is confirmed at surgery.

Unlike cerebral epidural hematoma, spinal epidural hematomas are usually venous in origin. Small epidural veins are torn with or without an associated vertebral fracture, though a hematoma in association with a fracture is more common. The hematoma may extend over several segments and, if large enough, can compress the cord, causing serious loss of function. Occasionally, such a hematoma presents as a chronic lesion at a time removed from the trauma. In contrast to the head, subdural hematomas are rare in the spine.

R. B. is hospitalized for some weeks until his cervical fracture heals. By that time little neurologic deficit can be found in his right arm.

Young B. S. is thrown from his horse as it jumps a hedge during a fox hunt. He becomes entangled with the reins and is dragged by the right arm at least twenty feet before his horse is stopped. He is brought to the emergency room with a dislocated right shoulder and a nasty gash on his head. The shoulder is reduced after radiographs reveal no fracture, and his scalp is sutured. A limited neurologic evaluation shows no focal abnormality, but he is quite confused and cannot recall his fall. A CT brain scan is compatible with brain contusion, and you admit B. S. for observation.

The next day he is much less confused but mentions that he cannot raise his right arm. You find definite muscle weakness and ask a neurosurgeon to see him. He confirms your impression of nerve damage. He suspects either a brachial plexus injury or a nerve root avulsion. Being an optimist, he schedules B. S. for a surgical exploration of the brachial plexus, but he asks you to order a myelogram first. What do you see?

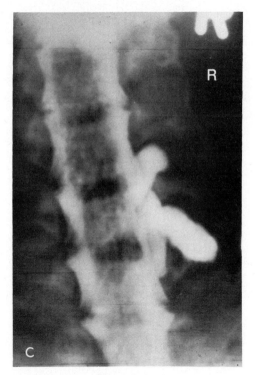

Figure 2-7c

Sadly enough, the diagnosis is obvious from the myelogram. On the left, the Pantopaque outlines normal nerve roots and root sleeves. On the right, two root sleeves are replaced by irregular sac-like collections of contrast. This is the classic appearance of nerve root avulsion. This cannot be corrected surgically and carries a poor prognosis.

Already fearing the worst, B. S. embarks on a course of physical therapy. When you next hear of B. S., it is in the society page. His wedding to a young woman from the physical therapy department has some tongues wagging.

Strange as it may seem, the very next day you are called to see A. S., a dirt bike rider, also thrown by his mount and dragged by his leg for about thirty feet through the desert. He is covered with dirt and painful cactus thorns. His thigh is ecchymotic and he cannot move it. Palpation and radiographs reveal a posterior dislocation of the left leg with a fracture of the posterior lip of the acetabulum. This is reduced, but A. S. continues to complain of pain and leg weakness, making you think of nerve damage. An EMG indicates damage to the left L4 root and you order a myelogram.

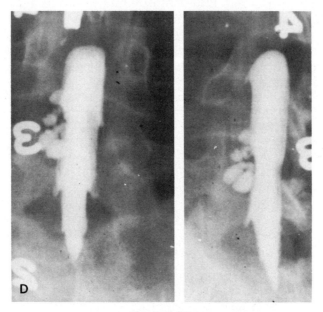

Figure 2–7d

Again, there are the characteristic findings of nerve root avulsion, with Pantopaque extravasation into irregular sac-like spaces replacing the L4 root sleeve.

Nerve root avulsion is the result of traction on an extremity, with separation of the nerve root at its origin from the spinal cord. This type of injury is common in the cervical region and, in the past, was a form of birth trauma caused by obstetric traction. Lumbar root avulsion is rare. Considerable force is required, and hip dislocation is a frequent concomitant injury. Myelography is the procedure of choice to diagnose this injury. Though all the patients illustrated in this section have had myelograms performed with Pantopaque, an oily contrast medium, water soluble metrizamide is also an acceptable myelographic agent and will be preferable in many patients.

D. S. AND C. G.

D. S. is a 27 year old construction worker who was helping a friend chop wood for the fireplace when the axehead flew off and struck him in the left neck, causing a deep laceration. His friend drove him to the emergency room while D. S. compressed the wound to staunch the flow of blood. When you see him, the bleeding has largely stopped. The sternocleidomastoid muscle has been almost completely severed and you can see the transmitted pulsation of the carotid artery in the depths of the wound. Physical examination is otherwise normal, and there are no neurologic deficits. Surgical exploration of the wound is undertaken, followed by closure of the laceration. Particular attention is paid to possible carotid artery damage. You conclude that the actual laceration did not reach the artery but know that the blunt force of the axehead could still have caused damage to the artery. After the surgical procedure is completed, you arrange for an angiogram of his left carotid artery. AP and lateral films from the angiogram are illustrated. What are your observations and concerns on reviewing these films?

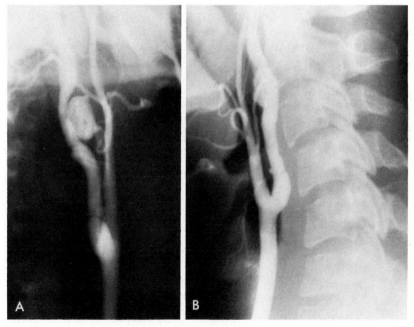

Figure 2–8a, b

On the AP film, the common carotid artery is normal. The external carotid artery lies lateral to the internal carotid artery and is also normal. There is an intimal flap near the origin of the internal carotid artery, which is also seen on the lateral film. It is the short fine defect in the contrast column. Above this flap the internal carotid artery is slightly narrowed for about 3 cm where another intimal flap is seen. This is indicative of a focal dissection. Immediately beyond the second intimal flap is an oval collection of contrast material that is clearly extraluminal.

This is a pseudoaneurysm. On the AP film, it is displacing and compressing the internal carotid artery. The internal carotid artery is irregular for two more centimeters, well above the angle of the jaw. Flow through the artery is not impeded by these traumatic changes, and an intracranial examination is normal.

After much debate, Mr. D. S. is treated conservatively, since he has no symptoms related to the carotid injury, and surgical repair would carry significant risk of inducing a neurologic deficit.

C. G. was riding with his wife along the Interstate when he suddenly stopped talking and slumped in his seat. She pulled onto the median strip and stopped the car. Blood was coming from a large ragged hole in his right neck. Shocked and not sure what to do, she was relieved to have the Highway Patrol pull in behind her. An ambulance arrives speedily and C. G. is brought to the emergency room less than 20 minutes after his injury. You find both a small entrance and a larger exit wound in his neck. The police tell you there has been a sniper shooting from overpasses on the Interstate where C. B. was hurt. More important, you find a dense left hemiparesis and can feel no right carotid pulse above the gunshot wound. Common carotid damage seems likely, and though the neurologic damage may well be irreversible, angiography is requested to confirm the clinical impression.

A single film from an innominate artery injection is demonstrated. What are your conclusions?

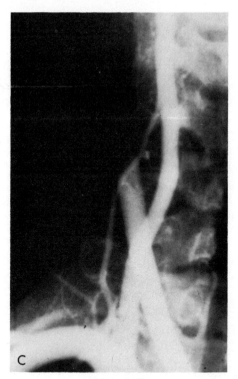

Figure 2–8c

The right common carotid artery ends abruptly at about the top of C5. The lumen at the end of the contrast column contains some filling defects, probably thrombus. No contrast medium is seen extravasating from the artery. Angiographically, it is not possible to evaluate the integrity of the arterial wall at or above the obstruction.

Surgical repair is undertaken and a small arterial rent and intraluminal thrombus are found. The intraluminal clots are removed and flow is reestablished. Mr. C. G. does not regain consciousness, however, and about six hours after surgery, the carotid pulse disappears again. He dies the next day.

Acute traumatic carotid occlusion is not well tolerated, and the initial insult may cause irreversible cerebral injury as in C. G. CT can be used to evaluate the intracranial effects of a carotid occlusion, but only angiography can demonstrate the injury itself. Such evaluation is important in patients like D. S., since bleeding from a lacerated artery or progression of a dissection with possible complete occlusion can occur at a time removed from the actual injury.

CASE 2-9:

R. T., M. L., J. R. K. AND L. D.

R. T., a careless weekend handyman, calls on Sunday to say that he has injured his left eye. When you meet him at the emergency room, he complains of severe pain, and you see he has a markedly injected conjunctiva and a minute scleral laceration. He was working with a lathe without wearing safety glasses, and a metal fragment struck him in the eye. Your inspection of the eye reveals no foreign body. You order some radiographs while waiting for the ophthalmologist to arrive. What do you see on these two views?

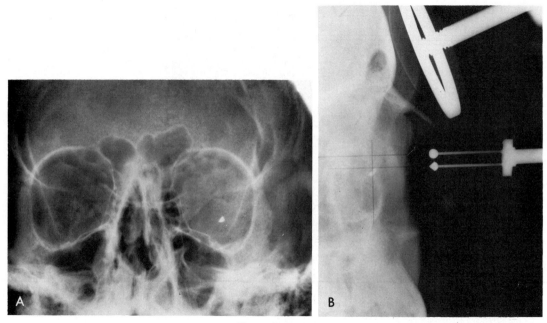

Figure 2-9a, b

There is a small metallic fragment seen on both views which is projected in the anterior aspect of the left orbit. This is useful information but does not give the exact location of the fragment relative to the globe. In the past, several geometric methods were available to localize the foreign body. Figure 2-9b is a film from a localization using the Sweet technique. These methods are only useful for radiopaque foreign bodies, are inherently limited by assumption of an average-sized globe and do not give detailed information about the relationship to various internal structures of the eye. In current practice, ophthalmologic ultrasound is the most useful tool for localizing foreign bodies, though CT scanning can also be used.

R. T. was fortunate that this fragment could be easily removed without complication or loss of vision. He vows to be more cautious in the future, but you have your doubts.

M. L., an aggressive young executive, comes in complaining of pain in the left eye and double vision. He was hit by a racquetball the previous evening and rapidly developed swelling and ecchymosis around his eye. This morning, he could not see clearly while shaving and noticed that his eye was actually protruding. Your physical examination discloses proptosis and limitation of gaze.

You order radiographs to exclude fractures, and none are seen. Because of the proptosis you order a CT scan to examine the orbital contents. What do you see on the single section illustrated here, which is through the inferior aspect of the orbit below the plane of the optic nerve?

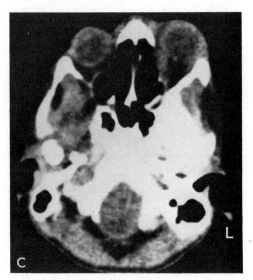

Figure 2–9c

The proptosis on the left is obvious. The globe is displaced forward by abnormal soft tissue seen along the medial orbital wall. This tissue compresses and displaces the orbital fat but is extrinsic to it. In view of the history, this is most compatible with an orbital hematoma. Such bleeding may be seen with or without a fracture and may be subperiosteal or actually within the orbit. Ultrasound is another method used to detect an orbital hematoma. Such hematomata usually resolve spontaneously.

M. L. does well with analgesia and cold compresses. In three weeks his eye is normal. He resolves to wear safety glasses while pursuing his favorite sport.

As you approach the emergency room entrance for your swing shift duty you see two young men approaching with clearly bruised faces. You wonder if there has been an amateur boxing contest but soon learn that the bashed up faces have occurred during a brawl at a rock concert. J. R. K. has his right eye swollen shut, and it is quite tender. L. D. has less swelling, but there is crepitance around his left eye. He has no problems with vision. Both are sent for x-rays of the facial bones. You see the films on J. R. K. first. What do you conclude from the two films shown?

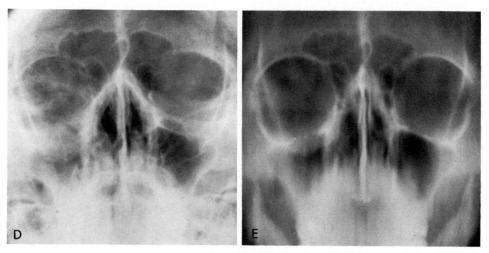

Figure 2–9d, e

There is soft tissue swelling over the right orbit and some streaks of air in the soft tissues. The right maxillary antrum is partially opacified, and there is a rounded soft tissue density where the orbital floor should be seen. You can compare this to the normal left side. The second film is a tomographic section that shows the blowout fracture of the orbital floor to better advantage. J. R. K. will have to be checked for visual problems caused by muscle entrapment when he can open his eye.

The films on L. D. are not quite as dramatic as those on J. R. K., and tomographs are not obtained. What are your observations? Where is his fracture located?

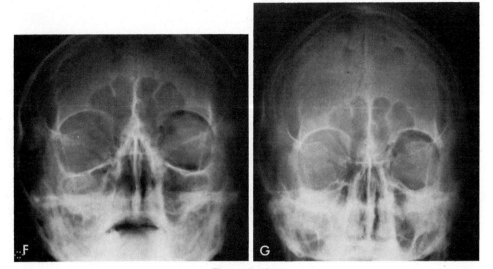

Figure 2–9f, g

The most striking finding is air around the globe. The left maxillary antrum is clear while the left ethmoid air cells are clouded, indicating that there must be a fracture of the medial orbital wall.

Aside from a spectacular black eye, L. D. has no problems, but J. R. K. does need surgery to restore full motion to his right eye, since the inferior rectus muscle was trapped.

When there is a blow to the eye, the force is transmitted to the globe and orbital contents, which can "blowout" the thin medial wall or the floor of the orbit. These two cases illustrate the radiographic findings of such injuries. If the medial wall is fractured, ethmoidal clouding and orbital emphysema are often seen. Orbital floor fracture is more significant, since trapping of orbital contents in the fracture may occur. This limits the motion of the globe and must be repaired if full eye function is to be maintained.

Facial bone films will generally demonstrate orbital fractures of the floor or lateral aspect. Tomograms may be needed for complete evaluation of these fractures. CT scanning with a high resolution scanner can provide detailed information in multiple planes and may be useful in some complex injuries.

CASE 2–10:

B. G. M.

At this point, this chapter makes a rather abrupt transition to the other structures in the neck. The esophagus and trachea can also be injured in both blunt and penetrating trauma and must be considered in this chapter. For the most part, injuries to the upper airway, trachea and larynx are not evaluated by radiography, though contrast studies may be needed to fully evaluate a perforation or a stricture. Films of the neck in a patient with a fractured larynx may show air in the soft tissue planes or disarrangement of the cartilages. The esophagus, on the other hand, frequently needs contrast study to look for perforations and also radiographs to locate foreign bodies. B. G. M. illustrates the first point.

Baby Girl M. had had a difficult intrauterine life because her mother was a very elderly primipara of 39 who developed toxemia at about 30 weeks. Careful monitoring brought the pregnancy to 36 weeks when a precipitous delivery occurred. B. G. M. was born through meconium and was rather vigorously suctioned after delivery. She had some respiratory difficulties shortly after suctioning, and the decision was made to intubate her. What happened during intubation was not at all clear except that the procedure was quite difficult. The respiratory difficulties improved rather rapidly, and there had been no significant meconium aspiration. However, B. G. M. does not feed well and runs a low-grade fever. It seems possible that the esophagus was injured during either the suctioning or the intubation just after birth, so you finally decide to do an esophagram. What do you see on this RPO supine film taken after the infant has swallowed a small amount of contrast material?

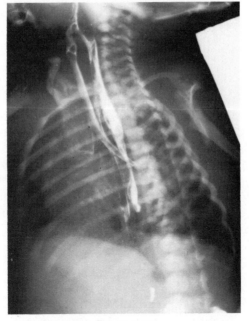

Figure 2–10

You can be excused for finding this film quite confusing. B. G. M. has aspirated some of the contrast material, which is filling the trachea and left mainstem bronchus. The esophagus is posterior to the trachea and contains only a small amount of barium. The important finding is the large irregular collection of contrast material seen behind the esophagus and trachea. This is first seen at the level of the lower cervical esophagus and tracks down the mediastinum nearly to the diaphragm.

At surgery, a small rent in the esophagus was found and repaired. B. G. M. escaped a serious mediastinitis, which is the most dreaded type of complication of such a perforation.

CASE 2–11:

MRS. I. G., R. S. AND LITTLE T. E.

Mrs. I. G., an obese housewife, calls you in an agitated state to say that she can't breathe and is choking. You arrive at her home and find that the problem is not respiratory but alimentary. It seems that she was a bit too eager this noon when eating chicken salad at her bridge club. She felt a sharp sensation in her throat as she swallowed a large chunk of chicken and then developed pain on swallowing and the sensation of something lodged in her neck. Over the next few hours, her apprehension increased as did her sense of choking. You drive her to the hospital and order a lateral radiograph of the neck. What is the problem?

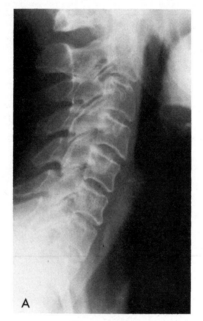

A

Figure 2–11a

Just as you suspect, the hapless woman has a fragment of bone lodged in the esophagus just anterior to the C6-7 intervertebral disc space. Do you see the calcification superior to this? That is ossification of the laryngeal cartilages and should not be confused with an opaque foreign body.

To evaluate the upper esophagus, you order an esophagram. As part of the examination, the radiologist has had the patient swallow a wisp of cotton soaked in barium.

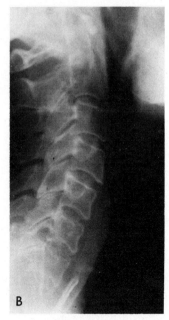

Figure 2–11b

The cotton has caught on the bony fragment. While not necessary in this case, this maneuver is useful in demonstrating the location of small or radiolucent foreign bodies in the esophagus.

R. S.'s mother practically drags the sobbing child into your office. It takes you some time to extract the problem from the angry mother and the crying child, but once you do, the problem seems simple. R. S. celebrated her fifth birthday yesterday and one present was a set of ten jacks and a ball. R. S. tried playing jacks, but the game was too complex for her and she shortly began to lose interest in the game. This morning, however, R. S. found a fun game. Instead of tossing the ball, she tossed the jacks; instead of catching them in her hand, her mouth was the catcher. Now there are nine jacks and R. S. has a sensation of something caught in her throat. You peer into her mouth and see no jack, so you order x-rays, glad that the jacks were metal ones. What radiographs do you request? What do you see?

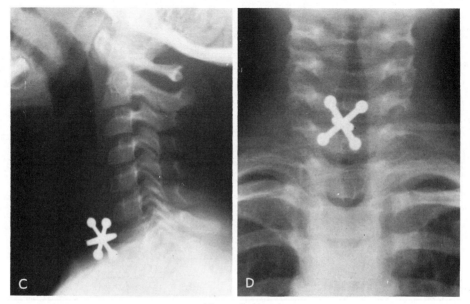

Figure 2–11c, d

With the history of something caught in her throat, the jack is most likely lodged in the high esophagus, so you have ordered AP and lateral views of the neck and upper chest. The jack is easily seen behind the tracheal air column at C7-T1 and is easily removed with the aid of an endoscope. R. S. really wants the jack, but her mother confiscates it and says R. S. must grow a great deal older before she can play with jacks again.

Little T. E.'s mother calls you out of a luncheon meeting. She is an excitable woman and is now on the verge of hysteria. It seems she came upon the child playing with her purse and claims she saw the child put a coin in her mouth, but when she got a look there was nothing to be seen. She is sure the child will choke and demands immediate action to find the coin.

Little T. E. shares her mother's excitement, and it is difficult to examine her, but a brief physical examination is normal. You order chest films. The PA and lateral films are shown. What can you tell the mother now? Is the coin in the trachea or esophagus?

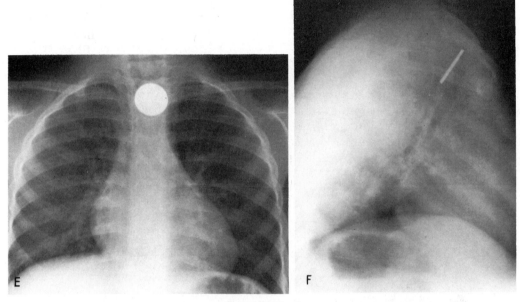

Figure 2–11e, f

In the frontal projection, the coin is seen en face at the level of the clavicles and on the lateral, it is seen on edge. This is the characteristic orientation of a coin lodged in the esophagus, reflecting the shape and orientation of the collapsed esophagus. Coins in the trachea will usually have the reverse orientation, since the tracheal rings are incomplete posteriorly and allow maximal distention in the anteroposterior plane. On lateral view, the coin is seen to lie posterior to the tracheal air column, a clear indication that the coin is not in the trachea.

After both mother and child are sedated, a Foley catheter is passed under fluoroscopic control into the esophagus beyond the coin. Gentle traction on the catheter after inflation of the balloon allows the coin to be delivered up into T. E.'s mouth and retrieved. Little T. E. goes home none the worse after a brief period of observation and richer by a trophy nickel.

CASE 2–12:

MRS. R. McK.

Mrs. R. McK. is an obese, accident prone woman who routinely gets every complication in the book. She was discharged from the hospital about two months ago after a prolonged stay brought on by a motor vehicle accident. She had skidded on an icy road, crashing into a large Sitka spruce at about 40 mph. Flail chest and aortic laceration were her initial diagnoses. She went on to develop adult respiratory distress syndrome and transient renal failure. A tracheostomy was placed to assist her ventilation after she had increasing problems with her endotracheal tube. It took weeks to wean her off the ventilator. She was discharged to a convalescent hospital where she stayed for eight weeks doing virtually nothing. At home for four days, she now complains of marked difficulty breathing, especially whenever she exerts herself. You examine Mrs. R. McK. and find little wrong except some noisy inspiration and expiration. Chest films show her healed rib fractures and surgical clips from repair of the aortic laceration. You suspect that her trachea is stenotic, and Mrs. R. McK. is so hefty that you decide to get tracheal tomograms. Even these are limited by her girth, so you obtain both AP and step oblique examinations. What do you think?

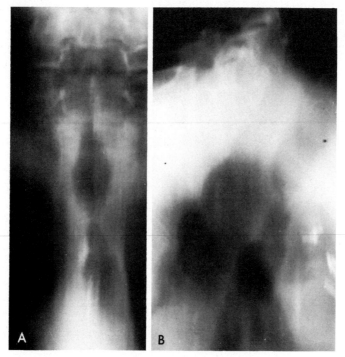

Figure 2–12a, b

There is a focal area of narrowing seen on both projections. The stenosis is quite discrete, and the tracheal lumen is about 5 mm in greatest dimension. The level of the stenosis is at the site of the end of the tracheostomy tube, which must have caused some irritation leading to the current problem. You are quite distressed by this event, since surgical repair of such stenoses is difficult and will be even harder in Mrs. R. McK. because of her recent surgery. You have some difficulty convincing the thoracic surgeon it must be done, but for once, Mrs. R. McK. breezes through surgery, has an easy convalescence and goes home breathing easily.

Tracheal stenosis may be seen in a variety of situations, including blunt and penetrating injuries to the airway. By far the most common cause of tracheal stenosis is the use of artificial airways, as in this case. It may be seen with both prolonged use of cuffed endotracheal tubes and following tracheostomy.

A variety of techniques are available to evaluate the cervical airway. While plain films will often suggest the abnormality, tomography is usually needed to fully define the narrowed segment. Xeroradiography may be very useful but is not universally available.

Contrast examination of the trachea can be done using bronchographic contrast if the simpler examinations do not provide a full evaluation.

CHAPTER
3

CHEST

The role of radiology in chest trauma is generally important. We will be evaluating this role in trauma to a wide variety of organs including the female breast, the lung and tracheobronchial tree, the esophagus, and the heart and great vessels. Especially important in this section will be blunt trauma which produces deceleration injuries, common in automobile accidents. The tracheobronchial tree and the esophagus are subjected to aspiration, inhalation and ingestion of solid, liquid and gaseous materials that damage tissues or cause mechanical obstruction. There is also the problem of intravenous injection of various materials that are carried to the lungs.

The wide spectrum of chest trauma demands a variable approach. Some problems will be resolved by evaluation of the standard chest radiograph. In others, more sophisticated studies will be needed. In some cases there will be ample time for cogitation; in others, prompt action will be imperative, especially in the setting of trauma to the heart and great vessels, flail chest, tension pneumothorax and complex, multi-system trauma.

CASE 3-1:

MRS. M. R. AND M. T.

The chest wall is subject to bumps and bruises, and the breast is especially vulnerable. While most trauma to the breast is minor, every now and then a problem in diagnosis will arise, as these two women demonstrate.

Mrs. M. R. had a right mastectomy for carcinoma three years ago and has had a mammogram of the left breast about once a year. She also regularly examines her left breast. She calls to say she feels a new mass but sounds so relaxed about it that you ask why she is not more concerned. She tells you she was struck by a squash ball and has a bruise where she feels the lump. She is sure the two are related. You ask her to come in for a check-up. Your physical examination does confirm the presence of a rather discrete lump in the upper outer quadrant of the left breast. It is somewhat tender and lies beneath an ecchymosis. Since it is near time for her routine mammogram, you suggest that Mrs. M. R. go to radiology and have the examination. What do you see on this lateral view?

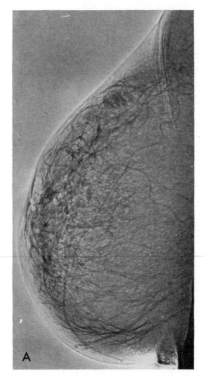

Figure 3-1a

The striking finding is a discrete, striated oval mass in the upper quadrant of the breast. No other change is seen from her earlier studies. This lump is not very ominous in appearance, though without the history of recent injury it would have to be approached as any solitary, palpable lump in the breast is handled. Instead, you ask Mrs. M. R. to return in two months for a repeat mammogram unless she feels that the lump is enlarging.

The radiologist calls you over to see the follow-up film. What do you think?

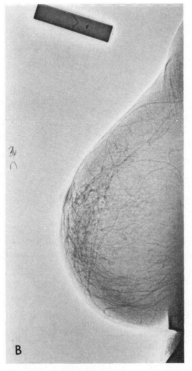

Figure 3-1b

The lump has completely cleared, leaving only Mrs. M. R.'s pattern of minimal ductal prominence, which has been present for several years. You are relieved, since all traumatic breast lesions do not resolve as completely or so fast. This one was most likely a simple hematoma and can be contrasted with the fat necrosis seen in M. T., your next patient.

M. T. presents a greater dilemma. She is currently 50. Her family history is strongly positive for breast carcinoma and, as a nullipara, she is individually at risk. Three years ago she was doing a final sprint after jogging when she ran into a lead pipe being unloaded from a truck. It struck her in the left breast, causing immediate pain and swelling followed by a rather awful black and blue mark. By the time the ecchymosis faded, a mass could be felt deep in the breast tissue in the upper outer quadrant. The mass decreased in size over the next few weeks, but then stabilized. A xeromammogram was obtained about three months after the injury. The lateral view is demonstrated. What is your impression?

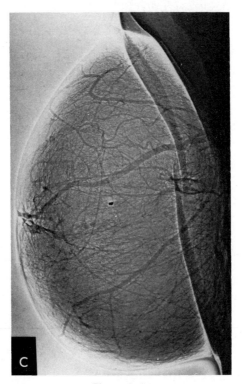

Figure 3–1c

Deep in the breast, almost against the chest wall, is an ovoid area of slightly increased density. The margins are quite easily seen, though there are some tentacles extending beyond the well-defined abnormality. This is the area of the trauma, and the breast is otherwise normal. One coarse ductal calcification of no clinical significance is seen. Long skin folds cross the mass. Under other circumstances, suspicion for malignancy would be rather high in a lesion with this appearance, but with the known recent injury in mind, traumatic change was felt to be more likely.

Both you and M. T. are somewhat nervous about the breast mass and follow it closely. It does not change in size over the next nine months, and a second mammogram is ordered. What is your conclusion now?

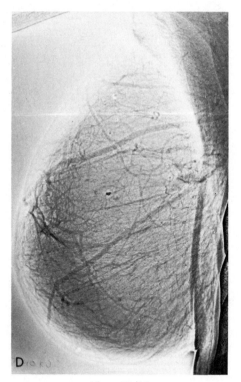

Figure 3–1d

The lesion is easily seen. Allowing for changes in mammographic technique and positioning, there is no significant change in the lesion. Your quandary remains the same. M. T. is becoming increasingly anxious about the lump, especially since another sister has just developed a breast cancer. Still, she will watch it longer if that is what you deem best.

The mass remains easily palpable over the next twenty months with no change detectable by either you or M. T. The stability of the mass is reassuring, but its continued presence is not. A third mammogram is performed almost three years after the injury. Technically, it is the best examination of the three. What do you see now?

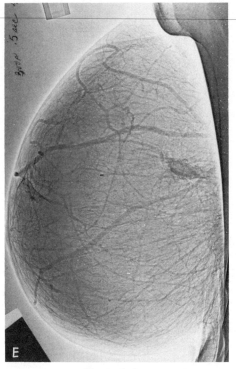

Figure 3–1e

There is no question that you would call the mass malignant with confidence if you were seeing the lesion without the history or previous films. As it is, all you can say is that there has been no change over nearly three years, which is unusual for carcinoma. Still, the very definite mass with irregular margins and spiculation is a disturbing picture.

By now, M. T. has had enough of watchful waiting. It is obvious to her that the mass will not go away on its own, and she is more than tired of worrying about it. When she pressures you to have it biopsied, you agree without much hesitation, since you had had the same thought.

The microscopic report is post-traumatic fat necrosis with fibrosis. M. T. is so happy to have this weight off her mind that she embarks on an extended trip to the Orient. You learn that she will get married at Katmandu, but you cannot make it to the ceremony.

Breast trauma is usually either minor or known to have occurred and, in general, radiographic evaluation in breast trauma is not indicated, but circumstances arise in which traumatic lesions are seen radiographically. Acute hematomas and swelling can appear quite ominous by mammography, and the correct diagnosis is aided by the history. As a rule, most traumatic changes regress with time, but residual scarring does occur in some instances. This residual disorganization of the breast tissue can give rise to areas that are indistinguishable from a neoplasm by current mammographic techniques. The proper approach to these problems must be selected on a case-by-case basis.

C. N. AND S. R.

Injuries involving the pleura can be quite confusing, especially when they are isolated or are discovered some time after the actual injury. Many of the x-ray findings, however, are characteristic of pleural lesions, as C. N. and S. R. illustrate.

Daredevil C. N. has just made a record high-altitude balloon ascent. Aside from a teeth-rattling descent during which he is snagged in a tree, he and the sporting press are delighted. Initially, he ignores the pain in his left chest, which began after he banged into the tree, but his wife finally forces him to come in to see you. Physical examination shows point tenderness of the posterior 6th, 7th and 8th left ribs. You suspect multiple rib fractures and order PA and lateral chest films. What do you see?

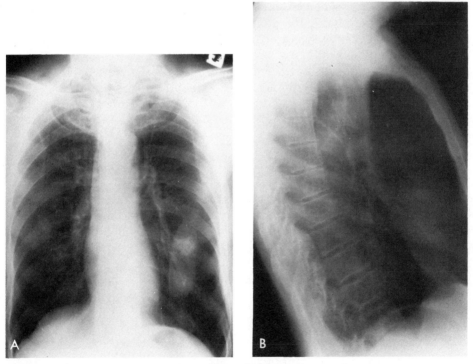

Figure 3–2a, b

On the PA chest, you see multiple rib fractures on the left at the levels you found to be tender. A more striking finding is the elliptical "mass" adjacent to the heart. A review of a film obtained several months ago is in order — was the "mass" present?

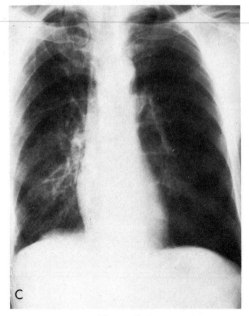

Figure 3–2c

This film is normal. Do you see the "mass" on the current lateral film? The lesion is lying far posterior, projected behind the vertebral column. It has a very sharp interface with the lung and makes an obtuse angle with the pleural surface. The lesion is longer than it is wide. These are all classical findings of an extrapleural mass. In view of the recent trauma, the most likely diagnosis is an extrapleural hematoma.

C. N. is treated conservatively, and follow-up chest films show decrease in the mass. When next you hear of him he is working on a midget submarine.

Significant bleeding caused by rib fractures occurs most commonly into the pleural space. Small extrapleural hematomas at the site of rib fractures are not uncommon, but oblique views may be needed to demonstrate them. An extrapleural hematoma of the size seen in C. N. is unusual and is presumed to arise from injury to the intercostal vessels with the bleeding confined by the parietal pleura.

S. R. comes to you complaining of left chest pain and low grade fever. On physical examination, there is dullness in the left lung base and you order a chest film. What do you see?

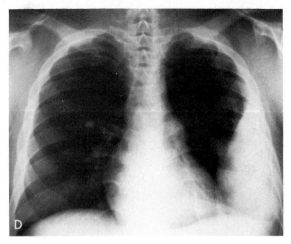

Figure 3-2d

There is a large opacity in the left base laterally. The shape, location and associated blunting of the left costophrenic sulcus are the findings of a pleural lesion, and you decide to order a decubitus film. Does the density change with position?

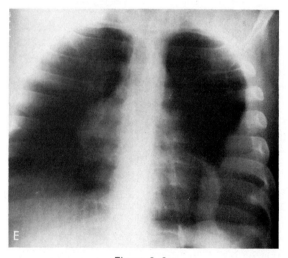

Figure 3-2e

There is no change, nor is there a free-flowing component. Fearing an empyema you call in a chest surgeon, who suggests a needle aspiration. When this produces what looks like altered blood and not pus, he is puzzled and asks S. R. about trauma. The young man at first denies any injury. When it becomes clear that surgical drainage is likely, he admits that three weeks ago he was injured by a large carton that fell against his left side at work. Since he is a probationary employee, he did not wish his employer to hear of it. At surgery, a large organized hematoma is found in the pleural space which requires local decortication.

A chronic, organized pleural hematoma such as this is not as common as a hemothorax, which is generally seen acutely and treated by tube drainage. The organized hematoma will mimic an empyema or neoplasm in its signs and symptoms as in this case, and a careful history is imperative.

CASE 3–3:

V. C., J. H. AND R. C.

V. C., a lady of the evening, is brought to the emergency ward by the police after an altercation with a "client." She was stabbed in the back with a switchblade that was found at the scene. Physical examination reveals a somewhat hysterical young woman with normal vital signs except for a tachycardia. There is a small wound in the left posterior fifth rib interspace. There is marked subcutaneous crepitation. On auscultation, breath sounds are diminished on the left, and a "crunching" sound is heard with each beat of the heart. A chest x-ray is obtained. What do you see?

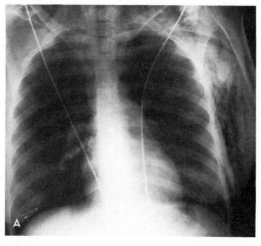

Figure 3–3a

There is marked subcutaneous emphysema in the chest wall and also a small apical pneumothorax, which is somewhat difficult to see because of the subcutaneous emphysema. There is a large pneumomediastinum. You can see air tracking lateral to the heart and also in the superior mediastinum extending into the neck. Between the left fifth and sixth ribs, there is a vague density in the lung. This is the result of pulmonary laceration and adjacent alveolar and interstitial bleeding.

While these findings are alarming, there is nothing that requires immediate action. The pneumothorax is small, and the pneumomediastinum is unlikely to be due to injury to the esophagus or a major airway, since the wound is peripheral. Most likely, it is due to disruption of alveolae, with tracking of air into the pulmonary interstitium. Air can then dissect into the mediastinum through the bronchovascular connective tissues. You decide to observe V. C. She continues to do well, and a repeat radiograph is obtained two days later. What do you see now?

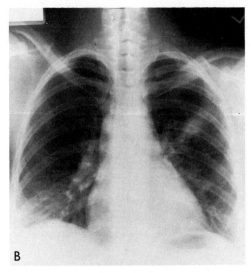

B

Figure 3–3b

The pneumothorax is no longer seen. The pneumomediastinum has also resolved, and subcutaneous emphysema is much diminished. The area of pulmonary parenchymal hematoma is larger and better defined and contains an area of central lucency, which is probably a pneumatocele, a cyst-like air collection.

Pulmonary hematomas may resolve completely after a few months or may leave an area of parenchymal scarring. They may also cavitate, forming pneumatoceles, which either resolve completely or persist as cyst-like, thin-walled spaces.

Were you surprised by the marked subcutaneous emphysema in this case? This is not infrequent in chest injuries. There is often a large pneumothorax that is the source of the chest wall air, but occasionally the pneumothorax is small or nonexistent, as if it had decompressed itself into the chest wall. You review the films on J. H. shortly after discharging V. C., and she emphasizes this point.

J. H. fell off her bike and came in complaining of pleuritic chest pain. On physical examination she is tender over the right ninth rib and has extensive chest wall crepitance. A minimally displaced rib fracture is seen on rib films. What do you see on the chest film?

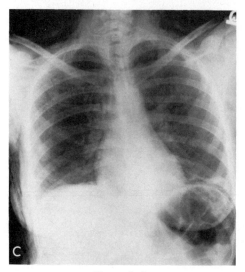

Figure 3–3c

J. H. has marked chest wall and cervical subcutaneous emphysema but no pneumothorax or pneumomediastinum. Clearly, the chest wall air is related to pulmonary trauma, but a pneumothorax need not be present.

A pneumothorax can be quite dramatic. Let's look at the case of Mrs. R. C. She is a sprightly 82 year old woman who seems to survive in the face of adversity. She has been admitted this time for repair of a ventral hernia and revision of her tracheostomy. Initial induction of anesthesia goes smoothly, but as the surgeon prepares to make his incision, Mrs. R. C. has a cardiac arrest. A couple of sharp blows to the chest are all that is needed to start her heart going again, but the anesthesiologist finds that breathing Mrs. R. C. has become much more difficult. A portable chest film is taken on the operating table. What do you see?

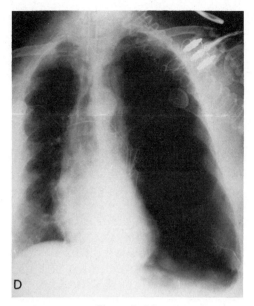

Figure 3–3d

The heart and mediastinum are shifted to the right, and no lung markings are seen in the left hemithorax. The left hemithorax is hyperexpanded, and the right lung is compressed. All these findings are those of a tension pneumothorax. A chest tube is placed on the left, and Mrs. R. C.'s vital signs return to normal. After some discussion her surgery is completed. When Mrs. R. C. is taken to the recovery room, a portable semi-erect film is obtained to check for residual pneumothorax and for the position of the chest tube.

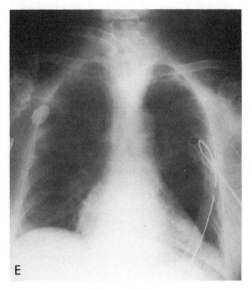

Figure 3–3e

All is well. The chest tube is in an appropriate position, and there is no residual pneumothorax. Mrs. R. C. is amazed at all the fuss and announces that she is leaving for a freighter trip through the Panama Canal in three weeks. And what's more, she goes!

The diagnosis of pneumothorax is generally not difficult, especially if upright films can be obtained. Although the air in the pleural space can be "trapped" anywhere in the pleural space, it will generally follow the dictates of gravity and seek the highest available space in the thoracic cavity and surround the lung. Therefore most small pneumothoraces are seen apically and laterally on the upright frontal film. The air contained in the pleural space is devoid of lung "markings" and is more lucent or "blacker" than the lung. It is delineated medially by a thin white line, the visceral pleura, made visible by air in the lung medial to it and the pneumothorax laterally. Small pneumothoraces may be studied using expiratory or decubitus films. Skin folds are sometimes confused with pneumothoraces, but they will disappear on repositioning the patient. Large bullae may be confusing because of their lucency and lack of markings but, again, the visceral pleural line characteristic of a pneumothorax is not seen. The walls of bullae are similar in appearance to the visceral pleural line but usually have a different orientation. A medial or basilar pneumothorax may not be identified because of the unusual location, but the radiographic findings are the same.

A pneumothorax implies a pleural laceration. The pneumothorax may increase with time, so even a small pneumothorax is important to diagnose. Large pneumothoraces and those under tension are usually clinically apparent, though the diagnosis should be confirmed radiographically prior to placement of chest tubes if there is time to do this.

Pneumomediastinum is diagnosed by the presence of air in the mediastinal tissue planes seen as "streaky" lucencies. These findings are often best seen on the lateral film of the chest. The mediastinal air, not infrequently, dissects into the neck and is more clearly seen there. The presence of a pneumomediastinum is also grounds for concern. While it usually arises because a lung injury allows air to enter the pulmonary interstitium, which then tracks into the mediastinum, the same mediastinal air may indicate injury to the tracheobronchial tree or the esophagus.

B. W.

B. W. was departing from a late night card party when he learned that a .38 caliber pistol always beats a straight flush. After being relieved of his winnings, he was shot and left to die. Fortunately, the noise of the shot brings help, and when he arrives at the emergency room he has revived and is quite agitated. He has an entrance would in the left mid anterior chest, but no exit wound is seen. An I.V. is started and a chest film is taken. A marker has been placed over the entrance wound. What do you see?

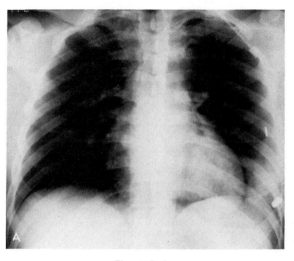

Figure 3–4a

The bullet has traversed the lung from above downward and now lies just above the diaphragm. There is an area of somewhat ill-defined density along the bullet track. This results from a combination of shearing, contusion and hemorrhage as the bullet gives up its energy in the lung. There is no pneumothorax or pleural fluid.

B. W. is admitted for observation, and his pulmonary injury heals without further difficulty. On the following page is a film taken one week later, showing marked improvement.

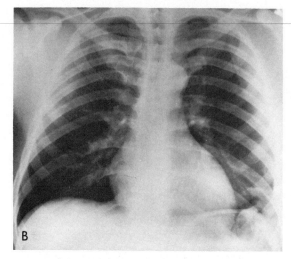

Figure 3—4b

The nature of a pulmonary injury caused by a gunshot wound depends on the caliber of the bullet and its velocity at impact. In general, the volume of tissue damaged does not compromise pulmonary function. There may be cavitation along the bullet tract. If the damaged tissue does not become infected, then complete healing of the lung or only minimal scarring is the rule. Hemorrhage or pneumothorax occurring at the time of injury may prolong healing.

J. D.

J. D., scion of a prominent local family, has a taste for gambling and fast women. He is stabbed with a long stiletto at the tables at Las Vegas by a jealous boyfriend while the showgirl in question watches. Rushed to a local hospital, he is found to have a tension pneumothorax, which is rapidly treated with a chest tube, partially reducing the pneumothorax. His family insists that he be transferred to your care.

He arrives by ambulance. You are confronted by a rather sullen young man and a bubbling water seal on the chest tube. Your next step is a chest film. What's wrong?

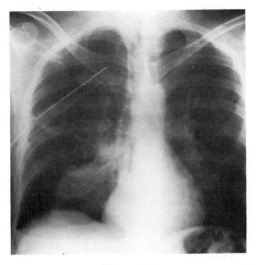

Figure 3–5

The chest tube remains in place and is in good position. There is, however, a large pneumothorax with an air fluid level. The right lower lobe is atelectatic, and the middle lobe is partially collapsed. Paralleling the spine, there is an unusual linear air collection, probably air in the mediastinum.

The continuous air leak and atelectasis as well as mediastinal air raise the possibility of injury to the tracheobronchial tree. This usually occurs in severe deceleration injuries during which the bronchi are fractured, but you recall the length of the knife used in this case and decide on immediate bronchoscopy. You find a laceration of the superior surface of the bronchus intermedius. Surgical repair is mandatory, upsetting J. D., but his father prevails on his scapegrace son to accept your decision. His postoperative course is rocky, but he pulls through and is taken to Monte Carlo to recuperate by his indulgent mother.

Tracheobronchial trauma must be suspected after either blunt or penetrating injury when there is persistent air leak, atelectasis or pneumomediastinum. The injury may involve central or peripheral bronchi and may have a delayed presentation. While there are other causes for these radiologic findings, if the diagnosis is not entertained and excluded, the results may be disastrous. When the transection is complete, the lung or lobe affected may sag away from the mediastinum or remainder of the lung when the patient is upright, an appearance that is highly suggestive of bronchial transection.

J. M. AND MR. E. H.

J. M. is an ill-fated 62 year old who is brought to your emergency room after being pinned between a bus and a truck. He was squashcd at about the waist and complains of abdominal pain when you first examine him. There are bruises over the epigastrium and lower thorax and diminished breath sounds, at the right lung base. You order some x-rays and ask J. M. for more detail about the injury while you wait. It seems he was squeezing between the tailgate of the truck and the bus. The truckdriver did not see him and started to move, lurching backward just a couple of inches, causing a quite substantial blow. The x-rays you requested are taken, and the chest film is the most interesting. What do you think?

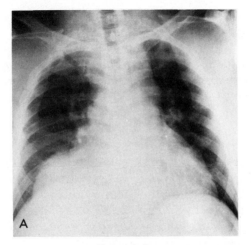

Figure 3–6a

There is a rounded elevation of the right hemidiaphragm medially. While you are wondering if J. M. has an acute diaphragmatic tear, the file room attendant brings in his old film jacket. On the following page is a film taken nine months earlier.

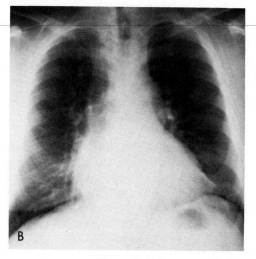

Figure 3–6b

Though the heart is enlarged and there are some chronic changes in the lungs, the right diaphragmatic contour is normal. Contrasting the two films, you feel quite sure that J. M. has ruptured his right hemidiaphragm and suspect he has herniated his liver through the rent.

Surgical repair is undertaken, and your suspicions are confirmed.

For many years, Mrs. E. H. has been trying to get her husband to come in for a physical examination. She finally succeeds on his 60th birthday. He looks to be in fine health and makes fun of his wife's concern. He has not seen a doctor in 35 years, does not remember that experience with pleasure and sees no reason to look forward to your physical examination. You take a clinical history and ask Mr. E. H. to get undressed. He grumbles but does do so.

The physical examination is normal except when you examine his chest. Breath sounds are diminished to absent over the lower left chest, and you think you hear bowel sounds. There is dullness to percussion in the same area. Further questioning does not produce any information to suggest lung disease. You order a chest film, which E. H. agrees to have after some argument.

Both the PA and lateral films are demonstrated. What is your interpretation of the findings?

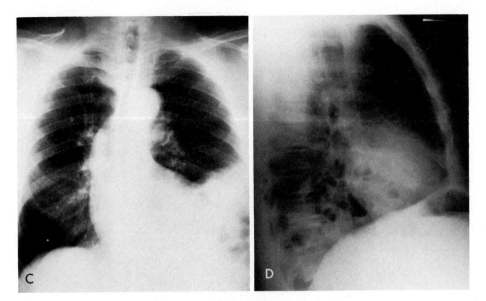

Figure 3-6c, d

The PA chest film is somewhat underexposed. Most of the film is within normal limits for the patient's age, but there is apparent elevation of the left hemidiaphragm with blunting of the costophrenic angle. On the lateral film, there are many rounded lucencies superimposed over the heart and posterior half of the thorax. The radiologist tells you that either the left hemidiaphragm is quite elevated or there is a tear in the diaphragm that has allowed bowel to herniate into the chest. Such a tear would probably be traumatic in origin, though congenital hernias may present late in life. Simple elevation of the diaphragm could be due to paralysis of the phrenic nerve, to an extensive eventration or possibly to a mass below the diaphragm.

Mr. E. H. has not given you any clue in his history, but you do remember that he last saw a doctor 35 years ago and that he found the experience distasteful. You decide to question him about that episode and any other medical encounters even more buried in the past.

Mr. E. H. is reluctant to tell you why he saw a doctor 35 years ago, but when his wife begins to tell the story, he interrupts. After he finished law school his family sent him on a European grand tour. He happened to be in Pamplona for the running of the bulls and, on a dare, joined the young men running before the charging animals. As luck would have it, he was unable to get out of the path of a bull and was tossed into the air and then trampled by the enraged beast. He awoke two days later in a Spanish hospital bruised and scratched. He was told he had had a concussion and was strapped up for several left rib fractures. The injuries healed rapidly, but the next letter from home told a terrible tale. His tossing and trampling had been captured by the movie news and was being shown all over the United States. For an ambitious lawyer, this was mortifying!

Mr. E. H. is reluctant to pursue what you feel is a diaphragmatic tear with bowel herniation that must have been present for 35 years. However, after he reads the series of articles you provide on delayed problems with these hernias, he agrees to further workup and possible surgery.

You do both an upper gastrointestinal series and a barium enema. One film from the barium enema is shown. What do you see?

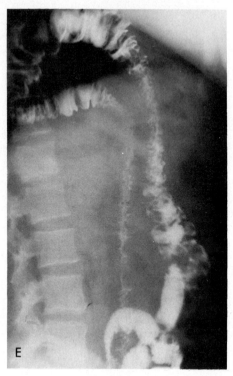

Figure 3–6e

The film is a lateral postevacuation film. The colon is clearly extending into the chest. The course suggests that it is passing through a rent in the diaphragm where the proximal and distal portions of the loop are approximated. The colon in the chest is not distended, suggesting no current obstruction. The GI series showed some jejunum in the chest, also not obstructed.

Mr. E. H. has his diaphragmatic tear repaired. All goes well, but you suspect it will be a long time before you see him without a writ of *habeas corpus*.

Diaphragmatic rupture may be a difficult diagnosis to make in the acutely injured patient. The mechanism of injury may be either penetrating trauma, in which the path of the injury should suggest the injury to the diaphragm, or blunt abdominal compression, such as occurred in J. M. When the abdomen is compressed suddenly, the diaphragm is torn by the increased pressure and deforming forces. This injury is more common on the left, and it is probable that the liver protects the right hemidiaphragm to some extent. Once a rent is created, abdominal contents tend to be drawn through by the negative intrathoracic pressure.

The radiographic findings will vary from subtle changes in the diaphragmatic contour to more obvious gross elevation with mediastinal shift away from the involved side. The presence of visceral gas shadows in the chest is, of course, very suggestive, but the herniated viscera may not contain gas initially. Upper gastrointestinal examination and barium enema will help if these structures are herniated, as will a liver scan if the injury is on the right. The use of intraperitoneal gas or intrapleural water soluble contrast may, at times, be helpful if the diagnosis remains uncertain.

As we have seen in E. H.'s case, the presentation of a traumatic disruption of the diaphragm may take many years. If bowel obstruction or incarceration occurs, these will bring the matter to medical attention. The findings may be noted on a routine evaluation of the chest, initiating further evaluation long after the occurrence of the trauma.

R. R. AND F. W.

R. R. is brought to the emergency room from the expressway where he had driven his car into a concrete abutment at high speed. The police cut him out of the wreck and discover he is fighting for breath and is slightly cyanotic. As his clothes are taken off it is clear that he has had major chest trauma, and part of his right chest wall moves asynchronously from the rest. You order an immediate chest film and call the chest surgeon. What do you make of this film?

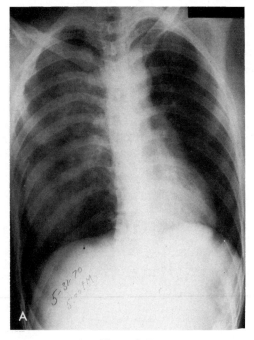

Figure 3–7a

There are many right rib fractures as well as a fracture of the right clavicle. There is also a large right tension pneumothorax with shift of the mediastinum to the left. A hazy density is seen throughout the right lung, most likely caused by contusion of the lung. The surgeon arrives and immediately places a right chest tube. R. R. improves but his respirations are still labored. It is clear that treatment of the flail chest is required, and so the ribs are strapped prior to endotracheal intubation for mechanical ventilation. Here is a film at the time of admission to the ICU just prior to intubation. What has changed?

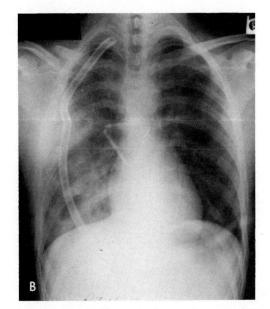

Figure 3-7b

The right lung remains hazy, but the pneumothorax is gone and the mediastinum has returned to the midline. The triangular metallic density is part of the chest support.

R. R. does well following these measures. Unfortunately, he is soon behind the wheel again.

Flail chest is clinically apparent and can only be suggested radiologically. Management is by stabilization of the chest wall, particularly "internal" stabilization by endotracheal intubation or tracheostomy and mechanical ventilation. The role of radiology in these patients is to demonstrate concomitant injury to the lungs, pleural and great vessels and to monitor the success of therapy.

   F. W., a retired dentist, decides to go out one evening to buy some ice cream. Unfortunately, this idyll is transformed into a nightmare when he is struck by a hit-and-run driver. Brought to the emergency room by ambulance, it is easy to see that he has sustained major chest trauma. He has no breath sounds on the right, has a flail chest with multiple rib fractures and there is marked subcutaneous emphysema.

   You order a chest film and call in a thoracic surgeon. What do you see on this semi-erect portable chest film?

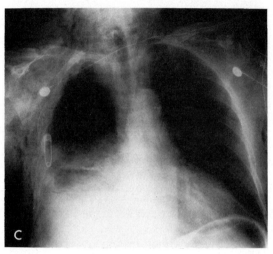

Figure 3–7c

   There is marked subcutaneous emphysema, multiple right rib fractures and a right clavicular fracture, all of which were clinically apparent. There is also a large right pneumothorax and the mediastinum is shifted to the left, indicating some degree of tension. There is a large right pleural effusion, undoubtedly blood.

   The chest surgeon arrives and, seeing the film, decides that the patient requires a chest tube and endotracheal intubation. These measures are accomplished with dispatch and F. W. seems to improve, but blood continues to issue from the chest tube, indicating continuous bleeding in the chest. You consider angiography to evaluate the great vessels, but the chest surgeon feels the situation is urgent and schedules an emergency thoracotomy.

   At surgery, the azygos vein is found to be avulsed from the superior vena cava. Resection of the clavicle is required to gain exposure, but the bleeding is then controlled. No other vascular injury is found. F. W. is then sent to the intensive care unit. Here is the postoperative film.

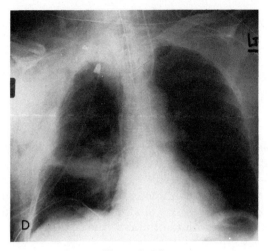

Figure 3–7d

The patient is intubated. Two chest tubes are in place, and the right lung is re-expanded. The density in the right mid-lung is residual blood trapped in the minor fissure, a pleural "pseudotumor." After a long convalescence F. W. is finally discharged.

Post-traumatic bleeding into a pleural space may come from the intercostal vessels, pulmonary vessels or major systemic vessels in the chest. This bleeding may be self-limited. The decision to employ angiography to localize and treat the bleeding vessel will depend on the clinical situation and the needs of the surgeon. Bleeding from intercostal arteries can be treated by embolization, while injuries to the great vessels must be surgically repaired.

F. W. has illustrated a vascular injury accompanying a flail chest. While vascular injuries often occur with other serious trauma, the next few cases will illustrate some of the wide variety of injuries that can occur to thoracic blood vessels with or without injury to other organs.

R. R., Jr.

R. R., Jr. calls your office on Tuesday and demands an appointment because his left arm has suddenly become swollen and discolored. R. R., Jr. is a spoiled, 22 year old son of a business tycoon who is not used to being told to wait his turn, so your receptionist is happy you have had a cancellation and can see R. R., Jr. in one hour. When he arrives, you see that his entire left arm is so swollen that his fingers look like sausages. The arm has a reddish-purple look, and the superficial veins over his shoulder are dilated. The only questions that remain in your mind are what made his axillary and/or subclavian veins thrombose and what can be done to decrease the swelling.

R. R., Jr. has a typical story. He is entering his 44 foot sailboat in the Hawaii race and had spent the entire weekend working on it. Sunday was very hot, and he worked most of the day on the rigging with his arms extended over his head. The sailboat is a passion with R. R., Jr., however, and it was only when friends arrived at the dock in the early evening that he realized he had not stopped for lunch and that he was very thirsty, hungry and tired. After he showered they went for dinner, but R. R., Jr. felt so tired that he left the party and went to bed at nine. When he awoke on Monday, his left arm was stiff and somewhat swollen. He thought it would get better, but instead it has gotten more swollen in 24 hours.

R. R., Jr. is annoyed when you tell him his condition is not uncommon and angry when you warn him not to expect a dramatic cure. You request a venogram to assess the extent of the thrombosis. The procedure is performed by placing a large needle or short catheter into an antecubital vein and injecting a bolus of contrast material. Films are taken over an extended period of time to demonstrate the level of occlusion and the collateral veins draining the arm. The first film shown is taken about five seconds after the start of the contrast medium injection. The second film is from a second filming series and was taken about 15 seconds after the start of the contrast medium injection. What do you see?

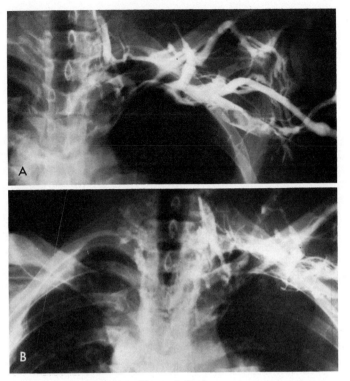

Figure 3-8a, b

The striking finding is the filling defect in the proximal axillary vein and left subclavian vein. This thrombus is not completely occluding the veins, but there is marked collateral flow through the veins over the shoulder. Some contrast material is reaching the neck, but the second film demonstrates that the venous drainage from the left arm is primarily by small collaterals in the neck and mediastinum. Retrograde flow in the left external jugular vein is present.

The degree of thrombosis, especially the medial extent of it, is greater than you had anticipated. R. R., Jr. is quite upset when you tell him that time and anticoagulation are all that can be offered. Also, he will have to give up any idea of active crewing in the Hawaii race. He blusters and demands a second opinion. When that is virtually identical, he storms out, but the next day his father's secretary calls for the prescription and instructions. Months later when R. R., Sr. comes in, he says Jr. is better.

Axillary and subclavian vein thromboses can occur following minor trauma and dehydration or after direct injury, or may develop spontaneously or in association with other diseases. Radiology has a limited role to play in these patients except to demonstrate extent of disease. Surgical intervention is rare, but when contemplated, venography is generally performed.

I. C. AND R. T.

I. C. is a brash, 22 year old motorcycle rider who lives in a fantasy world of Harley-Davidsons and motocross racers. One night when he is returning from a race, he sees two oncoming headlights, assumes they are two cycles and decides to split them apart. For reasons he can never explain, it does not occur to him, until it is too late, that two headlights usually mean a car. The impact hurtles him about 20 feet through the air, and he lands face down on the street. Initially, the only injury he feels is a dislocated shoulder, but when he tries to move, he finds that his left leg is broken. An ambulance brings him to the Emergency Room where examination confirms the leg fracture and also a posterior dislocation of his right shoulder. He has numerous abrasions, a probable nasal fracture and a tender anterior chest wall. Vital signs and breath sounds are normal. You request radiographs of I. C.'s right shoulder and left femur and also a supine chest film. The first two sets of films hold no surprises, but what do you think of the chest film? Why did you request it to begin with?

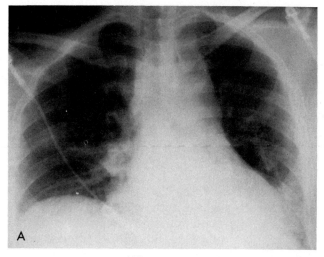

Figure 3-9a

You ordered the chest film because of the deceleration injury I. C. sustained. You are concerned about aortic transection. The chest film increases your concern because, even though the film is supine, the mediastinum is widened and its contours indistinct, especially on the left. You cannot make out the aortic knob or descending aorta, and the paraspinous stripe is widened. The left mainstem bronchus is depressed and there is fluid dissecting around the apex of the lung. This complex is classical for laceration of the thoracic aorta so you order an emergency angiogram. While the angiography suite is being readied, I.C.'s fracture is splinted. You explain angiography to him as he is wheeled into the angiography suite, and about 10 minutes later, you and the radiologist are standing at the film processor to see the first angiographic series. What do you see on this film taken during injection of contrast material?

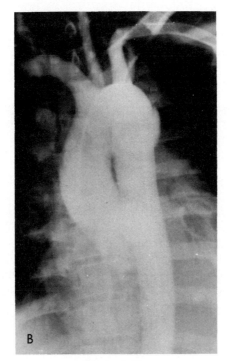

Figure 3–9b

The injection has been made into the ascending aorta. The origins of the brachiocephalic arteries are normal, but just after the origin of the left subclavian artery there is a bulge in the aortic contour and intimal flaps are seen. The picture is typical for aortic laceration and constitutes a surgical emergency. Generally, the adventitia is the only portion of the aortic wall that is intact. At surgery, the severed intima and media may be retracted as much as 3 or 4 cm. Delay in treatment often leads to sudden exsanguination.

As so often seems to happen, things occur in runs. You had barely finished with your motorcycle maniac when you are called to the emergency room to see an older man, who lost a race to a grade crossing with the commuter train he was trying to catch. R. T. is having trouble breathing and hurts every time he tries. He tells you he was going about 30 mph when he hit the train, and he figures he is still alive only because he was driving the largest car on the market. He broke the steering column when he hit it. You order a chest film expecting to find abnormalities associated with a combination of direct blunt trauma to the chest and a deceleration injury. Does the film support your hypothesis?

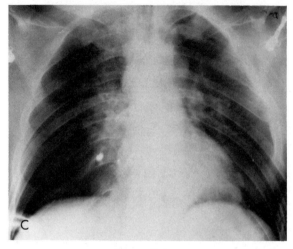

Figure 3–9c

R. T. is able to sit for his film. His heart is not enlarged, but it is hard to define the descending aorta or the aortic knob. The right perihilar area is obscured by a hazy parenchymal density, which you suspect is lung contusion. He has a whole series of left rib fractures with some pleural thickening. No pneumothorax is present, but there is some subcutaneous emphysema in the left axilla. A large metallic fragment is located in the tissues of the back, which R. T. tells you is from an old war injury. It led to one of his several Purple Hearts.

While the chest film is not typical for aortic laceration, the injury definitely is. You are concerned about the obscuration of the aorta and decide to get an aortogram on an emergency basis. Films from runs done in the RPO and cross-table lateral projections are illustrated. What do you see?

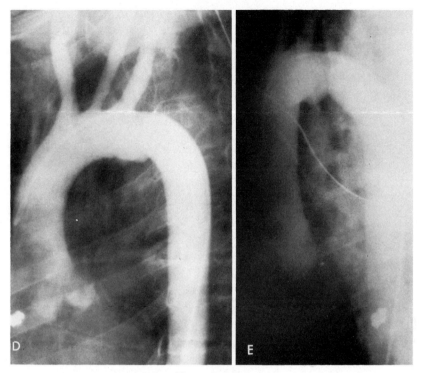

Figure 3–9d, e

The RPO is probably easier for you to interpret. There is an irregularity of the aortic contour immediately distal to the origin of the left subclavian artery, especially on the inferior surface, opposite the origin of the artery. A subtle intimal flap is also present. The lateral film also shows the contour deformity, and you call the operating room to let them know you have another aortic laceration and need to operate immediately.

R. T. does indeed have a complete transection at surgery. The operation is technically successful, but R. T. has a difficult postoperative course partly because of his many rib fractures, which keep him from breathing deeply. It takes him about four weeks to get ready for discharge and another month before he shows interest in buying a new car.

When angiography is performed in deceleration injury to evaluate the thoracic aorta, care must be taken to study the aorta from its root to the diaphragmatic hiatus, since tears can occur anywhere. Multiple projections may be needed to show the injury optimally. The most common site among survivors is just distal to the left subclavian artery, where the injury occurred in these cases. Brachiocephalic artery avulsions and lacerations also occur. The plain film radiographic changes are those of mediastinal hemorrhage secondary to dissection of blood through the damaged aortic wall. While these plain film findings may also result from venous bleeding, their presence mandates aortography to exclude the possibility of aortic laceration. The morbidity of aortography is greatly exceeded by that of an "expectant" approach to this situation. There is also a significant association of fractures of the first and second ribs and aortic laceration, probably as a result of the forces that must be applied to the chest wall to cause such fractures. Some authors feel that all patients with such fractures should have aortography.

T. F., a 34 year old man, is sent to you by a first aid station at the racetrack. He was a participant in a motorcycle race and has had a violent spill. As far as could be told, he entered a curve too fast, struck a bump and was thrown from his motorcycle, striking his right shoulder and chest on a barrier. He was shaken up but had no specific complaints. A chest x-ray was taken because of the deceleration injury. The x-ray unit at the first aid station is an older portable model and the resulting radiograph is somewhat limited but it was enough to prompt immediate ambulance transfer. What do you see?

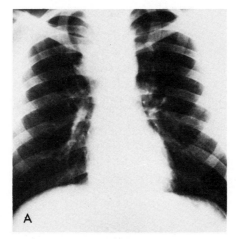

Figure 3–10a

The contrast of the film is so great that the lungs look black and there is no detail in the mediastinum. Remembering that T. F. is 34, however, the width and configuration of the superior mediastinum, which is especially full on the right, concerns you. The type of trauma makes you worry about injury to the thoracic aorta, and you also consider laceration of one of the brachiocephalic arteries or veins. The relative right-sided widening suggests innominate artery or superior vena caval injury. You should be wasting no time on speculation, since any arterial injury in this area has the potential for massive hemorrhage and death. You could repeat the chest film but, convinced that the mediastinum is abnormal, you go ahead with an aortogram.

Injection into the ascending aorta demonstrates that the aorta is normal in two projections, but there is a suggestion of a subclavian artery injury on the right. An injection into the innominate artery is then performed. What do you see on the arterial phase film on the following page?

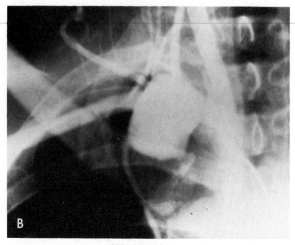

Figure 3–10b

There is a large collection of contrast material superimposed on the proximal portion of the right subclavian artery near the origin of the right vertebral artery. It displaces the internal mammary artery. This collection empties slowly, and several additional views do not demonstrate a neck. You conclude that this is a traumatic false aneurysm from a laceration of the right subclavian artery.

T. F. initially refuses any further therapy but returns about three weeks later because of vague distress in his shoulder. Surgery is performed, and the false aneurysm is removed. A rather short rent in the artery is easily repaired, and T. F. is soon back to cross-country motorcycle racing.

L. S. arrives at the emergency room in an ambulance with siren blaring and lights flashing. He lost a race with a trailer truck to an intersection and hit the truck broadside at about 60 mph, totally demolishing his car and killing his passenger. He has broken bones in his legs and left arm, is having trouble breathing and is barely conscious. His vital signs are remarkably good, however, and you set about evaluating these multiple injuries in a rapid but orderly fashion. A supine chest film is one of the first x-rays taken because of his respiratory problems. The superior mediastinum is very much widened, and there is bilateral apical pleural thickening, depression of the left mainstem bronchus and widening of the paraspinous stripes. These findings make laceration of the aorta likely, and emergency angiography is scheduled.

About one half hour after arrival, the angiographic catheter is positioned in the ascending aorta. The right femoral approach is used, and the radiologist carefully monitors passage of the catheter through the aortic arch. You are a little surprised when he says that he does not think there is an aortic laceration distal to the left subclavian artery, since this is the most common site of injury. The first film series is done in the AP position. What do you see on the single mid-arterial phase film shown?

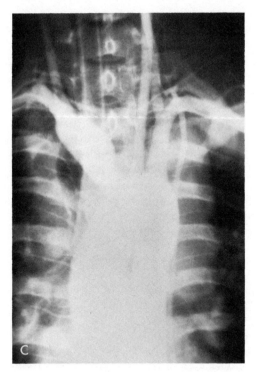

Figure 3–10c

The striking finding is the focal dilatation of the innominate artery. Subtle intimal flaps are seen both proximally and distally, so you know you are dealing with laceration of the innominate artery. On this film, the aorta itself seems normal but this projection does not adequately demonstrate the areas where tears most commonly occur, so the radiologist turns L. S. into the RPO position and does a second run, but it shows no additional injury.

Operative repair is decided upon and carried out in short order. Though the surgery goes well, L. S. has a left hemiparesis when he comes out of anesthesia. His multiple fractures provide an orthopedic challenge, but he finally leaves the hospital for a convalescent home with physical therapy expertise. He feels the whole episode has been most unfair. After all, if he had been two seconds faster, he would have beaten the truck.

Injury to the brachiocephalic arteries carries the twin dangers of massive hemorrhage and cerebral ischemia. Again, the diagnostic procedure of choice is angiography on an urgent basis.

CASE 3–11:

Y. D., W. R. AND G. W.

Y. D. is a 20 year old woman who is being evaluated for purpura and thrombocytopenia. Somehow when you do a sternal marrow biopsy your hand slips, and the trocar goes into the anterior mediastinum just to the left of the sternum. Though Y. D. has some pain, she is more alarmed by your reaction than by the accident itself. Her vital signs are normal and unchanging, and she has no trouble breathing. You accompany Y. D. to Radiology for a chest x-ray. What do you see on the PA and lateral films that were obtained?

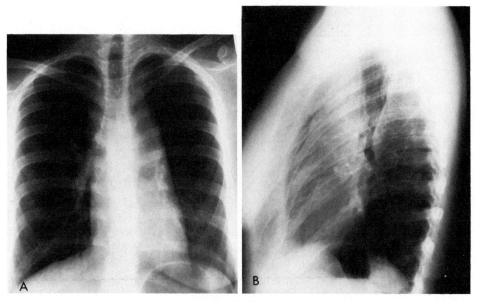

Figure 3–11a, b

The superior mediastinum is widened primarily on the left. The aortic knob is obscured, and there is a subtle added density with a straight margin superimposed on the left heart border on the PA film. No pleural effusion or pneumothorax is present. On the lateral film, there is an extensive density behind the anterior chest wall in the anterior mediastinum, extending from the manubrium to the lung base. This is all compatible with hemorrhage into the mediastinum.

Y. D. is quite all right as far as she is concerned but agrees to be admitted for observation. Nothing untoward occurs, and follow-up chest films are not alarming. A PA film taken three days after the accident is illustrated. What do you see?

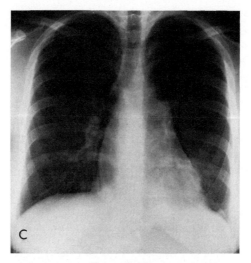

Figure 3–11c

There has been marked resolution of the anterior mediastinal mass. Now there is only a small left pleural effusion and some streaky atelectasis at the left base to remind you of your accident. As you suspected, Y. D. has idiopathic thrombocytopenic purpura and responds well to treatment. Fortunately, the bone marrow needle was short and did not enter any of the great vessels. All the same, Y. D.'s underlying illness led to formation of a large hematoma. Considerable mediastinal bleeding may occur without injury to the great vessels, as in this case when there is a bleeding diathesis or when there has been significant trauma. Damage to the great vessels must always be excluded angiographically if there is clinical concern.

Not all cases of penetrating trauma of the mediastinum will be so innocuous, as the next case will demonstrate.

W. R. is a 19 year old who wants to be a professional boxer. His trainers have high hopes for him, since he has natural ability and works out regularly. His major drawback is an uncontrolled temper, which gets him into innumerable brawls both within the gym and elsewhere. You encounter W. R. when he is brought to the emergency room by two friends following a pool hall confrontation during which he was stabbed in the left chest. The wound is about 1 cm in length and is near the midclavicular line just below the nipple. It is bleeding slightly and easily admits a probe for several centimeters. W. R. is feeling slightly faint, and you notice his neck veins are distended and his blood pressure is only

80/50. Chest examination is normal, but W. R. will not take a deep breath for you. You request a chest film, which is done AP supine because W. R. is rather shaky when sitting. Several possible diagnoses should pass through your mind at this point. Can you confirm any on this film?

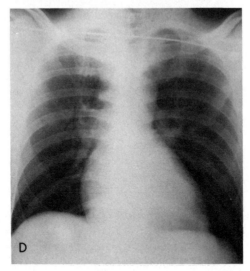

Figure 3–11d

Even though the film is supine, the cardiac silhouette seems large for a young man. The configuration is of no help. Adjacent to the left heart border, there is a paucity of lung markings, and with careful inspection you can tell there is a localized pneumothorax. There is also a wavy border or edge that projects over the heart shadow. The remainder of the examination is normal. You confer with the radiologist and conclude that W. R. most likely has an anterior mediastinal hematoma and a hemopericardium. The cardiac surgeon agrees and arranges for an emergency operation. A pericardiocentesis is done in the emergency room because of decreasing blood pressure. This produces 50 cc of blood and a startling improvement in the patient. At surgery, there is about 100 cc of blood anterior to the pericardium. A small pericardial rent and myocardial laceration are found and repaired. W. R. does well but leaves the hospital, vowing to get even with his assailant.

Pericardial tamponade is a clinical diagnosis, and radiologic evaluation should play a limited role in the acute situation. In W. R.'s case, the mediastinal hematoma was associated with injury to a deeper structure, the heart.

Cardiac injuries which are not immediately fatal may have few radiographic findings or they may be very dramatic. Consider the next patient, G. W.

G. W. is brought in from the freeway by ambulance, and a glance tells you that she is in very serious trouble. It seems she was driving a car involved in a high speed chase that ended in a crash at about 50 mph into a concrete divider. She was found semi-conscious in the front seat. Her major problem is respiratory, and you rapidly intubate her and request a chest film.

While you are waiting, a brief physical examination reveals large bruises on the forehead and over the anterior chest. There are coarse rales bilaterally and a loud mitral murmur. Nasotracheal suction yields copious pink, frothy material. The chest film is now available. What do you see?

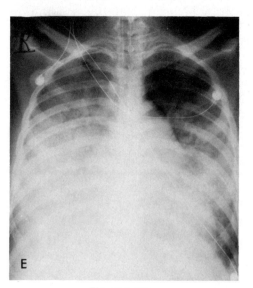

Figure 3–11e

There is diffuse bilateral alveolar consolidation with air bronchograms. There is no pneumothorax, pleural fluid or hemothorax. Though this is an AP film, the heart appears quite generous in size. Given the clinical history, there are several possibilities that you consider. The radiographic picture could be a massive aspiration, but there is no history or evidence of emesis, and the nasotracheal aspirate does not suggest this diagnosis. Massive pulmonary contusion or hemorrhage into the lung should be considered, but this would not explain her murmur. Pulmonary edema secondary to cardiac trauma seems to be the most likely diagnosis. In view of the loud murmur, the most likely diagnosis is disruption of the mitral valve.

G. W. is admitted to the ICU and responds only moderately to medical management. An emergency cardiac ultrasound is performed, and it shows abnormal motion of the mitral valve. Cardiac catheterization confirms the diagnosis of the free mitral regurgitation. G. W.'s congestive failure becomes intractable, and it is decided to replace her mitral valve. At surgery, the anterior papillary muscle is torn, as is the anterior cusp of the valve. After a stormy postoperative course G. W. is finally discharged, but into the care of the police.

The heart may be injured in both penetrating and blunt thoracic trauma. With high or low velocity penetrating trauma, cardiac injury is usually readily apparent because of the path of the wound and the dramatic clinical picture. Blunt trauma affects the heart in a variety of ways. There may be myocardial contusion with subsequent dysfunction or arrhythmia. The forces applied to the chest may be great enough to cause disruption of the myocardium, either the free wall of the heart or the ventricular septum. The cardiac valves or subvalvular apparatus may be ruptured, causing valvular incompetence.

Conventional radiology contributes relatively little to the evaluation of cardiac trauma. The cardiac contours may be evaluated, and the secondary abnormalities, such as pulmonary venous hypertension or pulmonary edema, may be seen. Detailed evaluation will require more sophisticated studies: cardiac ultrasound and catheterization.

G. F. AND M. K.

G. F., an unfortunate housewife, is cleaning the storage closet when she knocks over a shotgun, which discharges. The blast catches her at close range and virtually blows her right leg off. Fortunately, the neighbors hear the noise and scream and summon help. She is brought to the emergency room in profound hypovolemic shock. Immediate fluid resuscitation is instituted, and she is readied for the operating room. On the way to the operating room, a routine chest radiograph is obtained, which is normal.

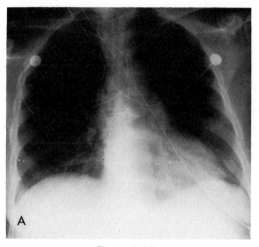

Figure 3–12a

After a long surgical procedure requiring vascular and nerve repairs it looks as if G. F. has a slight chance to keep her right leg, and she is sent to the intensive care unit. Twelve hours later you are called by the ICU resident, who reports that G. F. became agitated and dyspneic and has developed hypoxia. You request another chest film and return to the hospital. What do you see now on the film on the following page?

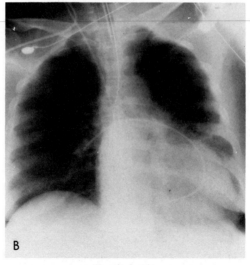

Figure 3–12b

Your initial impression is that there has been little change from the earlier film. A Swan-Ganz catheter and an endotracheal tube have been placed and are in satisfactory position. Closer inspection reveals scattered patchy areas of air space opacification and a diffuse increase in the interstitial lung density. Aspiration or massive pulmonary embolus could produce this clinical and radiographic picture, but you feel the findings are best explained by the adult respiratory distress syndrome or "shock lung." In spite of appropriate therapy, G. F.'s hypoxia increases, and higher pressures are required to ventilate her. Here is the morning portable film thirty-six hours after admission. What now?

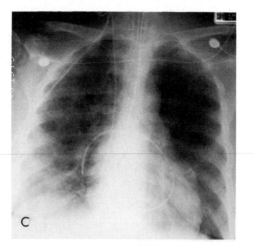

Figure 3–12c

The diffuse air space filling is much more extensive and confluent than on the previous film. There are no pleural effusions. Careful observation reveals some reticular lucencies in the lung that do not correspond to the bronchial tree. This is interstitial air, which means that the pressures required to ventilate G. F. are now high enough to cause alveolar rupture. Four hours later you are paged to the ICU. G. F. has suddenly deteriorated. The obvious thought is that she has a pneumothorax. A chest film confirms this.

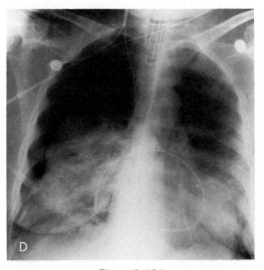

Figure 3-12d

Rapid placement of a chest tube relieves the pneumothorax, but G. F. continues to have a stormy course, with superimposed sepsis requiring a three week stay in the ICU. Ultimately she does go home and miraculously her leg was saved, though it is several inches shorter than the left.

Adult respiratory distress is a clinical entity with many causes, including infections, thoracic and non-thoracic trauma and shock of any etiology among others. Clinically it is characterized by progressing dyspnea and hypoxia beginning twelve to twenty-four hours after the initial insult to the patient. There is refractory hypoxemia secondary to intrapulmonary shunting and diminished compliance of the lung. Radiologically the syndrome includes diffuse alveolar infiltrates, which may be quite asymmetric at the outset but generally progress to uniform, bilateral confluence. These are due to loss of fluid into the alveoli, hyaline membrane formation, and peripheral atelectasis.

While survival is possible, the patient is not infrequently left with markedly abnormal lungs, as in M. K., your next patient.

Miss M. K. was a young woman who planned to have a home delivery of her first child. She had lined up a good midwife, but she was alone when she went into premature and very precipitous labor. She decided she could handle the delivery herself and all went reasonably well until after the child was delivered. Miss M. K. suddenly felt insecure and called the midwife who arrived about twenty minutes later. She found M. K. in shock, lying in a pool of blood. She called an ambulance and bundled up the baby. There was no evidence that the placenta had been delivered.

Miss M. K. responded to fluid and blood replacement, but she had a series of complications of both the delivery and the period of hypotension. The placenta had to be delivered, and there was a severe perineal tear that had to be repaired. Uterine atony with further bleeding occurred. She developed acute renal failure that lasted eleven days and adult respiratory distress syndrome, which required prolonged endotracheal intubation and ventilator therapy. It took weeks to get her back to unassisted ventilation, and at that point her lungs looked like a battlefield. How would you describe them?

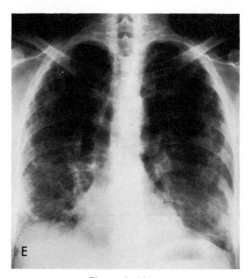

Figure 3–12e

The lungs show extensive fibrosis. The upper lungs bilaterally are hyperlucent and have many bullae. Circulation has been redistributed to the lower lungs because of the destruction in the upper half of the lungs. Miss M. K. does eventually go home, but she is severely limited in her exercise tolerance and finds care of the baby almost more than she can handle.

One day you get an emergency page and are told that she is being brought in because she can't breathe and is turning blue. By the time you reach the emergency room, she has been intubated and a portable chest film is being taken. You hear no breath sounds and M. K. is indeed cyanotic. Breath sounds are markedly diminished bilaterally and the chest is tympanitic. You order chest tubes, sure of what the film will show and, in fact, place an 18 gauge needle on the right and hear a confirmatory rush of air. The film arrives. What do you see?

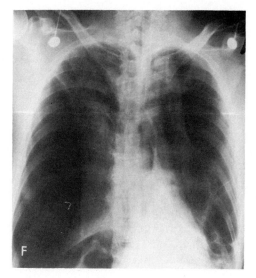

Figure 3-12f

There are bilateral tension pneumothoraces with little residual expanded lung. Ironically, some lung cannot collapse because of adhesions. Bilateral chest tubes do expand the lungs, but Miss M. K. develops an overwhelming pneumonia and never leaves the hospital. A coughing fit apparently was sufficient trauma to cause the bilateral pneumothoraces in her damaged lungs.

CASE 3–13:

B. B.

When B. B. moved east to Oyster Bay he wanted to be popular, and so he decided to establish himself as an athlete. He told everyone in his high school that he was a champion swimmer at Santa Barbara High, even though the only sport in which he excelled was suntanning. His bravado led him to refuse a life jacket while sailing on Long Island Sound, and so today when his sailboat capsized in a sudden squall, his companions ignored his cries for help, taking them for a joke since he was such a great swimmer. The crew of another boat finally realized he was in genuine trouble and fished him out of the water. By that time he was unconscious and blue. He is brought to the emergency room about 30 minutes later and you order a chest film. What do you see on this AP film?

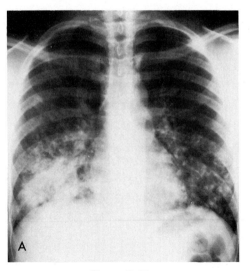

Figure 3–13a

There are infiltrates in both lung bases, and they are much more prominent on the right than on the left. The heart is normal, and no other abnormalities are seen.

The laboratory reports a normal blood count, and B. B. is afebrile. He is now conscious, is coughing and has rhonchi at both lung bases. Everything is consistent with a near drowning, and you expect B. B. to recover rapidly. Though rather upset by his accident, he does just that and you order a follow-up film prior to discharge 72 hours later. What do you see?

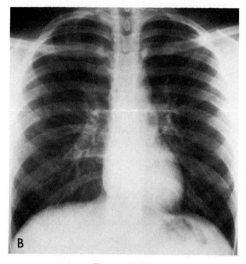

Figure 3-13b

This PA film is normal. Such rapid clearing is typical of near drownings of this nature. The air space consolidation seen in drowning or near drowning is due to either residual aspirated water or edema fluid in the alveoli from injury to the pulmonary tissue. This is rapidly cleared unless there is superimposed infection or some other complication of the drowning.

R. H. AND G. F.

Little R. H. is brought in by his somewhat remiss mother. It seems that this morning, while she was entertaining a gentleman friend, the little rascal got into some cleaning fluid. She thinks he may have drunk some since, though a little was spilled, more seems to be gone from the bottle. The boy did vomit once after she found him. Now he has started to cough.

You hear rales in both lung bases and decide to get chest films. What do you see?

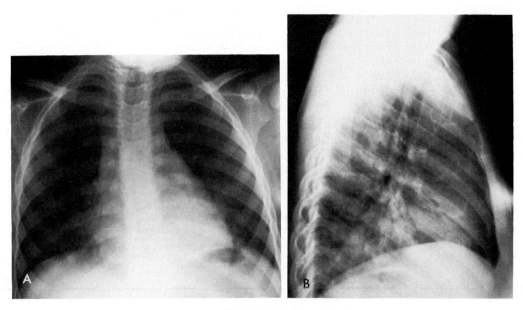

Figure 3-14a, b

There is air space filling at both bases, particularly on the left where there is dense consolidation. You hospitalize R. H. for observation. Two days later another set of films is obtained. What now?

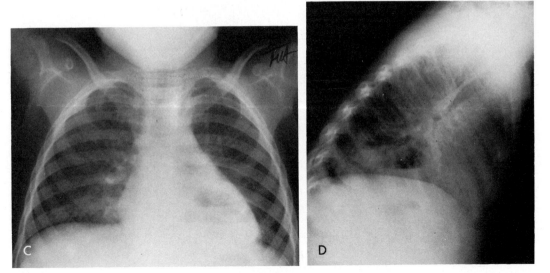

Figure 3–14c, d

The infiltrate in the right base is now more extensive. Did you see the small radiolucencies within the area of infiltrate on the right, or were you too busy admiring the large air fluid levels that have shown up on the left? These are pneumatoceles and are common in hydrocarbon-induced pneumonitis. Little R. H. does well and is discharged before his infiltrates are completely cleared. These may take several weeks to disappear, and Mrs. H. does not keep her follow-up appointment.

The mechanism of pulmonary injury in hydrocarbon ingestion is not entirely clear. The ingested hydrocarbons may be aspirated during swallowing or during emesis or may reach the lungs through the blood stream after absorption from the stomach. The radiographic changes often take several hours to develop. This phenomenon is not limited to children, as your patient G. F. illustrates.

G. F. is your gardener and has come to do the lawn but, as has often happened, he has forgotten the gasoline for the mower. To avoid your wrath he decides to siphon some from his truck. Shortly thereafter he runs into your office, sputtering that he has swallowed a mouthful of gasoline and is sure he will die.

You reassure him but after he cuts the grass, he comes back with a variety of complaints. You examine him and hear rales in the right lung base. Again, a chest radiograph seems in order. What do you see on the film on the following page?

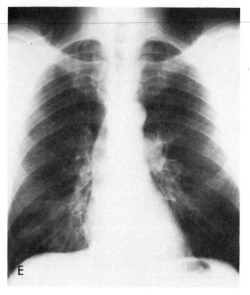

Figure 3–14e

There is a hazy, ill-defined density in the right base. You decide to observe him for a while, and so four hours later another film is obtained.

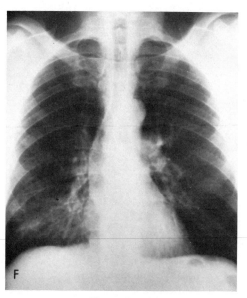

Figure 3–14f

On this radiograph, the density is slightly more extensive; G. F., however, feels well and somewhat sheepish and decides to go home. A week later he is back to do the lawn, is fine and has a bright new gas can.

B. L. is one of several people brought to the emergency room after rupture of a tank of chlorine gas at his job. His breathing is labored, and he has diffuse, moist rales. He is agitated and has a tachycardia. A chest film is obtained on the way to the ICU. What do you see?

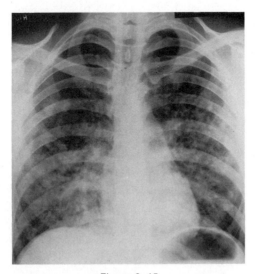

Figure 3–15

There are bilateral, patchy and confluent areas of air space consolidation, most marked in the lung bases and perihilar areas. As you expected, B. L. has pulmonary edema caused by the diffuse chemical injury to the lung. The edema increases over the next few hours, causing severe hypoxia that requires ventilator therapy, but B. L. does eventually recover without significant loss of pulmonary function.

Chlorine is only one of many gases used in industry that pose a danger of diffuse lung injury if inhaled. Some of these agents can produce severe damage to the airways, resulting in permanent disability or death even if the patient survives the initial insult. The initial radiographic manifestations will depend on the concentration and duration of exposure, but diffuse air space consolidation is common to all these injuries. A similar radiographic picture occurs after smoke inhalation also because of pulmonary edema.

M. I.

M. I. is dropped off at the city dispensary by two young men who say he overdosed on heroin. They disappear before any questions can be asked, and your attention is turned to M. I., who is unresponsive and has labored breathing and tightly constricted pupils. Blood pressure is about 80 systolic. There are a few needle marks on one arm. You think a heroin overdose is indeed likely and so you administer a morphine antagonist, with a rewarding improvement in M. I.'s condition. As he comes around, his statements are confused and inappropriate, bordering on psychosis. He insists he must, and will, die and no one will be able to stop him. "Quicksilver has seen to it." Physically, there seems to be little wrong with M. I., but you draw blood for drug levels and decide to get a chest x-ray. You also request aid from the crisis clinic.

The chest x-rays are shown. What is your diagnosis?

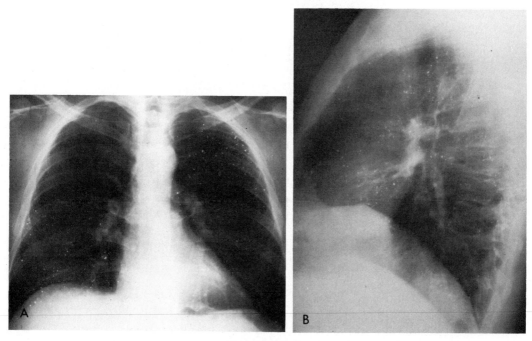

Figure 3–16a, b

The reference to quicksilver should now be quite clear. There are innumerable small, round metallic densities scattered throughout the lungs in a vascular distribution. You are sure M. I. has injected metallic mercury intravenously.

A while later, the crisis clinic doctor summarizes what he has learned. M. I. had become depressed over the past few weeks after the death of his brother in a skydiving accident. Sure the death was his fault because he had packed the parachute, he decided to atone by suicide.

The mercury had been injected several days earlier, and he was counting on a slow death from chronic mercury poisoning. He had also injected other substances, and the heroin was a first-timer's overdose.

You turn M. I.'s care over to the crisis clinic personnel. Some months later you hear he is doing well.

Metallic mercury is clearly visible in the lungs after an intravenous injection. Most other substances that are injected intravenously will not be as visible on a radiograph, though their distribution will be similar. The x-ray will be normal in some instances but may show patchy infiltrates and cavitary lesions in others, particularly if there is associated infection.

S. B. AND LITTLE A. C.

S. B. is brought in by his concerned mother. It seems that he and his brother were squabbling over possession of a toy pellet gun and S. B. put all the pellets in his mouth so his brother couldn't use them. That was a week ago and now the boy has fever and a persistent cough. The boys can only find five of the six pellets. Mrs. B. feels that the boy must have swallowed the missing pellet. You have another idea and order a chest film. Does this confirm your suspicion that S. B. aspirated the missing pellet?

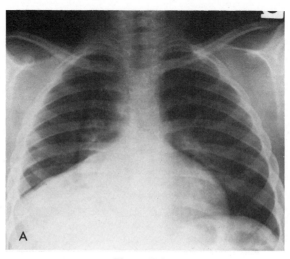

Figure 3–17a

There is atelectasis of the right lower and middle lobes with depression of the right main bronchus and hyperinflation of the right upper lobe. There is no mediastinal shift. The history and radiographic findings are both strongly suggestive of foreign body aspiration, and you hospitalize the child for bronchoscopy.

The missing pellet is found in the bronchus intermedius and retrieved with some difficulty. S. B. is soon back home ready to engage in further mayhem.

Mrs. C. brings in little A. C. to see you because of a cough that has been going on for over two weeks. She says the child has also had intermittent fevers. On physical examination the most striking finding is a loud wheeze over the left chest. What are you thinking of?

In a two year old such as A. C., an aspirated foreign body should be a strong consideration, and so you decide to get a chest film. What do you see?

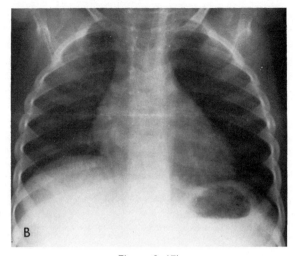

Figure 3-17b

On the frontal film, there is a rather subtle difference in the radiographic density of the two lungs. The left lung is more lucent than the normal right lung. No infiltrate is seen. This suggests air trapping in the left lung. What other views might confirm this impression?

An expiratory view of the chest would clearly demonstrate air trapping, but in children it is often impossible to get such a film. A left lateral decubitus view was obtained instead. In the decubitus position the dependent lung will normally be in expiration. What about it?

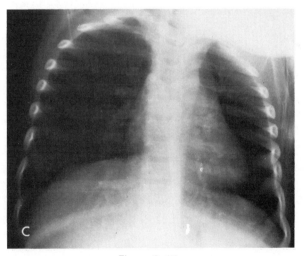

Figure 3-17c

In this left lateral decubitus view, the left lung remains inflated, confirming your impression of air trapping. You question Mrs. C., and she says she is always very careful about small toys and nuts. Little A. C. chimes in that Daddy always buys sunflower seeds at the movies and he loves them. Mommy is mean because she doesn't give him nuts!

Sure enough, an intact sunflower seed is recovered from the left mainstem bronchus. Little A. C. is fine when you see the family the next day but his dad looks sheepish and his mom, somewhat triumphant.

Aspiration of a small toy or nut or other food object is not uncommon in children. The event may be forgotten or the child may not be able to tell his parents about the problem. Radiographic evaluation can be very helpful, especially if there are no focal findings on physical examination or the idea of an aspirated foreign body is not being considered clinically. As we have seen, there may be either air trapping or atelectasis secondary to the foreign body in the airway, depending on the airway's reaction to the presence of the foreign body. Most aspirated foreign bodies are not radiopaque. Expiratory or decubitus films can be exceedingly helpful in the demonstration of subtle air trapping.

MRS. L. J.

Mrs. L. J. had all her teeth removed before she was twenty. She has never found dentures comfortable and over the years has become quite good at eating without her teeth in place. This habit causes trouble when she swallows large, unchewed pieces of food, and she has had to be esophagoscoped to remove chunks of meat several times. At her fortieth birthday party she is eating a piece of fried chicken breast when she does it again. L. J. continues to eat for a while but then feels choked and unable to swallow. When the party ends, she phones you and you meet her in the emergency room. Both of you agree she has food stuck, and an endoscopist is called in. She removes food from the mid and distal esophagus, and when a large piece of chicken is encountered at the gastroesophageal junction, she feels she has reached the real culprit. It does not dislodge easily, and when she pushes it into the stomach, L. J. has chest pain. Both of you are concerned about esophageal laceration, since the discomfort increases. A nasogastric tube is passed without difficulty, and you request a chest film. What do you see?

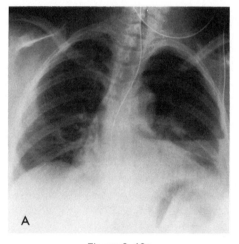

Figure 3–18a

Mrs. L. J. is listing to the left and has taken a rather poor inspiration. There is a long air fluid level in the left hemithorax as well as obscuration of the left hemidiaphragm and subsegmental streaky atelectasis in the left lower lobe. There is a gas collection beneath the diaphragm, which should raise the question of free air in the abdomen.

Quite concerned about esophageal laceration with its associated problems of mediastinitis, you request an esophageal swallow with water soluble contrast material to demonstrate the site of the leak.

Two spot films from this study are illustrated on the following page. What do you see?

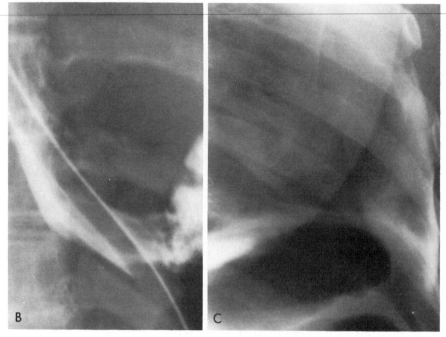

Figure 3–18b, c

The initial film shows contrast material in the esophagus. Just proximal to the gastroesophageal junction, it changes course, entering the left hemithorax through a tear about 2 cm in length. The second spot film shows the contrast medium flowing freely in the pleural space.

Mrs. L. J. tolerates surgical repair well and, while in the hospital, you have her fitted with new dentures, hoping to avoid further problems. She finds the new set comfortable and uses them regularly.

Esophageal laceration is a serious complication of ingestion of a foreign body or a large chunk of food and subsequent attempts to remove the impacted material endoscopically. The level of the esophageal laceration will be determined by the level of impaction or technical factors affecting the instrumentation. An esophageal laceration is a possible complication of all esophageal instrumentation, including simple intubation or endoscopy as well as dilatation of strictures or removal of foreign bodies.

Penetrating thoracic trauma may rarely involve the esophagus. Severe blunt trauma to the chest can also cause a transmural tear and, of course, the Boerhaave syndrome is an esophageal tear caused by the trauma of repeated retching or vomiting. Esophageal tears may be asymptomatic at occurrence but usually cause pain. Chest films may show mediastinal air or enlargement and pleural effusion. These changes are generally seen in the left or are more marked on the left. Contrast studies are performed first with water soluble contrast media as a rule, but if this is normal, barium may be used to look for a subtle leak. In general, early recognition of a tear decreases morbidity.

CHAPTER 4

ABDOMEN

INTRODUCTION

Abdominal trauma takes many forms. Radiology has little role to play in some injuries and will be quite important in others. For example, clinical suspicion of splenic rupture can be evaluated radiographically, aiding in the decision to operate on the patient or to observe him. Foreign bodies that have been swallowed can be located, and the progression of scarring from acid ingestion is easily followed radiographically. On the other hand, patients with high velocity penetrating injuries generally go straight to surgery, and radiology will play only a minor role in early assessment of the injury. Such patients may require more extensive radiographic evaluation later in their hospitalization.

The challenge for the radiologist is to meet each of these unpredictable and sudden events with efficiency and logic so that appropriate therapeutic actions may be taken expeditiously. Each patient will be a little different from any other, and choice of procedures will depend on these variations. The multitude of procedures available to study splenic injury, for example, are illustrated. Reasons for choosing one approach over another in a given patient will be discussed. Hard and fast rules on how to approach these patients are not really possible. Rather, the radiologist and referring physician need to know what tests are available and which one to use in any given circumstance.

CASE 4–1:

L. G.

L. G., a flamboyant, middle-aged man, is well known to you and his friends for dramatic gestures, so no one reacts when he says he is going to commit murder. The reason for this threat is the desertion of his wife, who is planning to marry a younger man. You personally feel you should have listened more carefully when you receive a phone call from the emergency room that L. G. has been shot. It seems that he did threaten the boyfriend with a gun and was somehow shot in the ensuing struggle.

L. G. has an entrance wound with powder burns in the left midaxillary line about the level of T8. There is an exit wound near midline in the abdomen an inch above the umbilicus. He is bleeding from both wounds and is having trouble breathing. You set several things in motion. The operating room is notified of an emergency thoracoabdominal exploration; intravenous lines are placed, blood is drawn for crossmatching and other laboratory data, a portable chest film is taken and Mr. L. G. is monitored for vital signs. When the chest film demonstrates a sizable left pneumothorax, a chest tube is placed, which eases his breathing.

Within 20 minutes of L. G.'s arrival in the emergency room, he is taken to surgery. The bullet track is explored through a thoracoabdominal approach. Damage to the left lower lobe and diaphragm is repaired. The spleen is intact. Four holes in the splenic flexure of the colon are closed, and two in the stomach are found and repaired. The abdomen is thoroughly irrigated, drains and a diverting colostomy are placed and Mr. L. G. is closed and sent to the recovery room. All goes well for about 10 hours and then a nurse calls to say she is getting very bloody fluid back from the nasogastric tube. Vital signs remain stable. When you see Mr. L. G. about 10 minutes later, he is vomiting up large quantities of blood and clots. You are reluctant to reoperate but realizing it may be necessary, you consider the options available. Watchful waiting with blood replacement is one approach. Endoscopy seems unlikely to be successful because of the vomiting and carries added risk and difficulty because of the very recent surgery. Mr. L. G. stops bleeding spontaneously for a few hours, delaying need for action, but then bleeds massively again and his vital signs become unstable. Surgery becomes inevitable unless the bleeding can be stopped. You decide on angiography both to demonstrate the site of bleeding and for treatment with vasoconstrictors or embolization if feasible. Three films from the celiac angiogram are shown. The first one is a preliminary film after the catheter has been positioned. There are some pertinent observations to be made. What do you see?

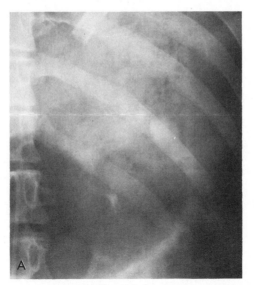

Figure 4–1a

The stomach is quite distended. The mottled pattern in the cardia is typical of blood. There is an oval density superimposed over the eleventh left rib that is not in the kidney, which is lying lower. What is this?

While you have not been shown a film taken before any contrast material was injected, this density was not present. You should be suspicious that it is extravasation of contrast material at the bleeding site. Do the next two films from the angiographic series confirm this? What exactly is bleeding?

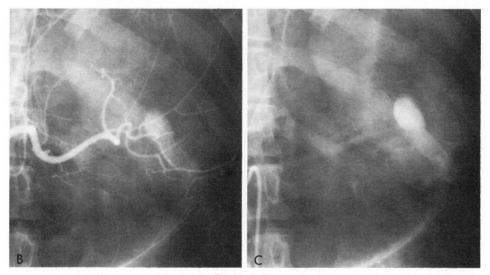

Figure 4–1b, c

The collection is quite distinct on the venous phase film. It does not have the characteristics of bleeding into a viscus, since it is discrete, does not outline mucosal pattern and stays in one place. On a single run, you would be hard put to locate precisely where the bleeding is, but you do know that it is coming from a branch of the splenic artery; since you also know blood is being aspirated from the stomach, you suspect a short gastric artery. Oblique runs support this conclusion. The bleeding must be either in an ulcer crater or intramural because of its discrete nature. It is on the posterior surface of the stomach near the greater curvature. Vasopressin infusion is unsuccessful in controlling the bleeding, and embolization is not likely to succeed without jeopardizing the splenic circulation. Mr. L. G. continues to bleed, so you return him to the operating room.

At surgery, his stomach is filled with blood and clots. There is a large submucosal hematoma near one of the bullet holes that had been closed and a small mucosal rent, which is bleeding briskly. Hemostasis is easily obtained, and the operation is rapidly completed. You conclude that a small artery must have been transected or lacerated by the bullet and gone into spasm. As the spasm relaxed over time, the hemorrhage started.

Mr. L. G. does well medically, but charges have been made against him because of his actions. His wife decides that if he agrees to a divorce, she will drop the complaint. This lifts L. G.'s spirits, and he is soon pursuing the nurses.

R. M. AND S. B.

R. M. is a 35 year old man who intervened in a barroom brawl just as one of the combatants drew out his switchblade knife. The resulting stab wound was in the left lower quadrant. Realizing what had happened, the two brawlers joined forces, beat up R. M. and ran. The police arrived soon thereafter and called an ambulance, and poor Mr. R. M. is brought to the emergency room. Though bruised in body and soul, he is quite reluctant to have anything done. His biggest complaints are pain at the stab wound site and in the right flank where he was kicked. When he sees that his urine contains blood, he becomes somewhat more cooperative. You are more concerned about the stab wound than about the hematuria, but you request an intravenous urogram and it excludes serious renal injury. You then explain the risks of stab wounds and the problems in determining their depth on clinical grounds. Mr. R. M. finally agrees to have an injection of contrast medium into the stab wound to see if the contrast medium enters the peritoneal cavity. Knowing that false negatives can occur, you are a bit reluctant, but decide it is as far as R. M. will let you go.

A radiopaque tube is positioned in the wound and a preliminary film is taken.

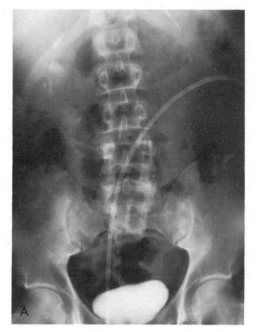

Figure 4–2a

Contrast medium is seen in the kidneys and bladder. Bowel gas pattern is within normal limits. The catheter tip is seen at the left of the abdomen. You see no free air and an upright film taken during the urogram had also not shown any. You inject dilute contrast material through the catheter under fluoroscopic control. Mr. R. M. is fascinated by what he sees. Two films taken after the injection are shown. The first is an AP film; the second is LPO. What can you tell Mr. R. M.?

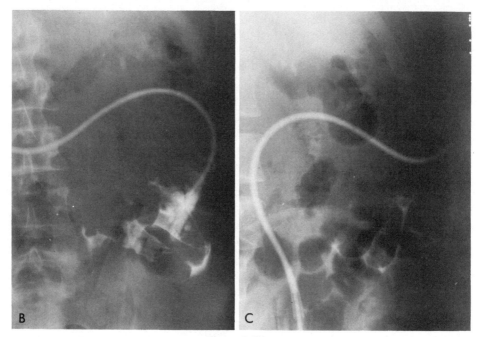

Figure 4–2b, c

Contrast medium is surrounding small bowel loops and is dispersing throughout the abdomen, indicating that the stab wound does enter the peritoneal cavity. Some contrast material remains in the abdominal wall, but this is unimportant. False negative wound tract injections can occur when the injected contrast material does not follow the injury tract but instead dissects in the abdominal wall. Fortunately, the procedure here gives a clear-cut answer.

Mr. R. M. wants neither exploration nor observation for his injury. Actually, his risks are rather low, since bowel tends to move away from low velocity penetrating instruments and no solid viscus is likely to have been injured. After a long discussion you get him to promise to return if there is any problem and to make an appointment with you in one week under any circumstances. When you next see him all is well, except you discover that R. M. is already suing the bar where the injury occurred and is considering suing the ambulance company for losing his tie. You wonder if you are next.

You are still thinking about the problems of the clinical evaluation of stab wounds when S. B. is brought into the emergency room accompanied not only by the ambulance crew, but also by the police.

It seems that S. B. is a 20 year old unemployed high school dropout who has been trying to make a living in the drug world. He is not very clever, and when he is warned off a territory, he pays no attention. The police found him left for dead in a gutter and bring him to the emergency room when they feel a pulse. Your examination reveals several stab wounds to the abdomen, but otherwise S. B. is not seriously hurt and you suspect he fainted when attacked. It is not even clear that any of the stab wounds enter the peritoneum, since the majority are definitely quite superficial. Once again, you resort to injection of the stab wounds that seem deepest. An abdominal film taken after the first injection is demonstrated. What do you see?

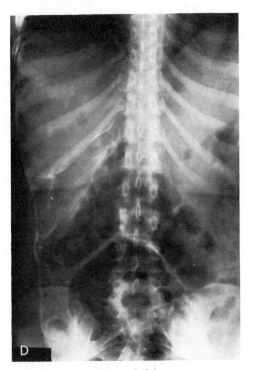

Figure 4-2d

Contrast material is seen in the right paracolic gutter, outlining the lateral and inferior margins of the liver.

You are amused at the relief S. B. exhibits when you request that he remain in the hospital for observation, although he is dismayed at the prospect of a possible exploratory laparotomy. Apparently, the street is too warm for him at present.

Though two stab wound injections have been illustrated here, you must remember that false negative examinations occur with some frequency. Also, a positive examination does not give any information about injury to either hollow or solid abdominal viscera. These limitations are important considerations in utilization of this procedure.

CASE 4-3:

P. W., MRS. C. M. AND MR. M. G.

P. W. is an 18 year old college student who has recently taken up riding unicycles as a lark. He is good at it, but as his skill increases he keeps trying taller cycles and does fall on occasion. He shows up in your office one afternoon looking a bit haggard and bruised. When you get him into an examining room, he tells you he just can't keep any food down. He vomits within minutes of drinking or eating anything. The problem has been going on for about two days, first with nausea and then with some vomiting. Today nothing will stay down. He says he doesn't have time to be ill because he is riding in a college circus in three days and there are lots of rehearsals he must attend.

You suspect you know P. W.'s problem. You ask about new unicycles and recent falls and get the expected answer. He has had really bad falls recently and took quite a header three days ago. Somehow he lost his balance and his seat simultaneously and landed in a heap on the cycle. The most painful part of the fall was a handlebar in the gut, which knocked the wind out of him momentarily.

What is your working diagnosis and what radiographic examination do you order? Two films are demonstrated. Do they support your diagnosis?

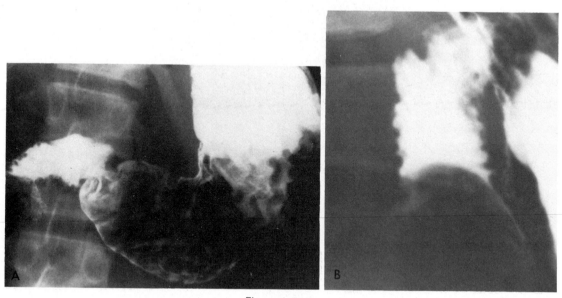

Figure 4-3a, b

The examination you order is an upper gastrointestinal series. The striking finding is a smooth, well-demarcated mass obstructing the duodenum in its second portion. The mass seems to be intramural and is in a typical place for a traumatic intramural hematoma of the duodenum. This was your working diagnosis, and you tell P. W. it is unlikely that he will be performing on Saturday. You hope the hematoma will resorb without surgery, but only time will tell.

Duodenal hematomas can occur without trauma in anticoagulated patients and in some blood dyscrasias. These hematomas may occur anywhere in the duodenum. They are often diffuse and may have a "stacked coin" appearance. Traumatic duodenal hematomas usually occur in the fixed, retroperitoneal part of the duodenum, as in this case. Many of these respond to conservative therapy, but others will require surgical intervention. P. W. was lucky. He did miss the circus but was eating solid foods in less than a week after the diagnosis was made.

⊂⌇⌇⊃

Both construction and demolition fascinate Mrs. C. M., a 70 year old widow. Since her retirement she has spent hours being the premier sidewalk superintendent at large building projects around the city. Construction crews find her interest amusing but are fond of her and often tell her when something of special interest will occur. She rewards them with Tollhouse cookies and cinnamon buns. Some of the men are beginning to be concerned about her because she has been unsteady in recent weeks, tripping over broken paving and bumping into barricades. Recently, when the last piles were being driven for a large building near the waterfront, Mrs. C. M. brought champagne to celebrate the end of this stage of construction. While watching the final piling go in, she lost her balance, stumbled and fell forward, striking her mid abdomen against a low barricade. She was shaken up but insisted on going on with her party. One of the crew took her home, and they all worry when she does not appear the next day. In fact, it is over three weeks before she reappears and they hear what happened to her.

The morning after her fall she had no appetite and vomited her orange juice. Her stomach really hurt. She went back to bed, but by afternoon she felt even worse and went to see her doctor. He admitted her to the hospital when he discovered that her abdomen was very tender where she had struck the barricade. He also heard for the first time about her unsteadiness.

On admission Mrs. C. M. had an abdominal series, looking for fluid, free air, masses and abnormal bowel gas pattern, since her doctor was worried about the blunt trauma. The supine film from the series is illustrated on the following page. What do you see?

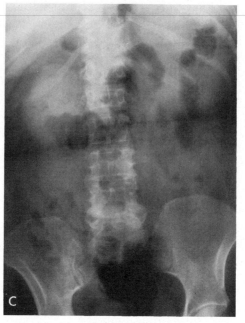

Figure 4–3c

The only abnormality is some slightly dilated and edematous-appearing small bowel in the left upper quadrant. The valvulae are just a bit thickened, which makes you wonder if C. M. has a small bowel injury. Certainly there is no evidence of free fluid, and no masses are present. Neither the spleen nor the liver is enlarged. The right kidney is easily seen and looks normal. The left one is obscured by the overlying bowel.

Mrs. C. M. continued to have pain during the night. Laboratory data are not helpful except there is some blood in her stool. Intravenous fluids are started, since she vomits when she eats, and an upper gastrointestinal series is ordered for the morning. One film is illustrated. What is your diagnosis?

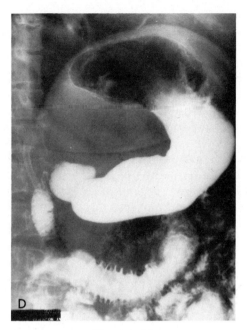

Figure 4–3d

The thickened small bowel that was seen on the abdominal series is jejunum. It is somewhat dilated and, by now, the valvulae are quite thickened. The stomach and duodenum are normal, as is the remainder of the small bowel that was seen on other films of the small bowel. The diagnosis is diffuse submucosal bleeding into the proximal jejunum, which should respond to conservative therapy.

Mrs. C. M. does well, and her doctor uses her hospitalization to look into her increasing unsteadiness. New glasses solve that problem easily. He had worried about transient ischemic attacks or Meniere's disease and is relieved to find a simple solution.

The construction workers are pleased to have her back and relieved that nothing very terrible has happened. They present her with a gardenia and construct a small observation booth for her where she will be safe and sheltered. She provides Tollhouse cookies and cinnamon buns in profusion.

Shortly after Mrs. C. M. is back at her sidewalk superintendent post, Mr. M. G. comes to your office because of abdominal pain that has been present for several days. On examination you find he is tender in the left upper quadrant and has blood in his stool. At 30, he is rather young for carcinoma, diverticula or ischemic disease, and so you are somewhat at a loss to explain his pain. You question him more carefully about his recent activities, hoping for a clue. When Mr. M. G. tells you that he has just become a window washer for a downtown skyscraper, you ask if he has had any job-related injuries. At first, M. G. says no, but then he remembers that about a week ago a cable slipped and he was thrown violently against the safety railing of his platform. He then realizes that his abdominal pain developed after that event.

You order a barium enema and are not at all surprised by the findings. What does this single film show?

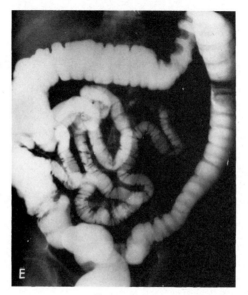

Figure 4–3e

The colon is normal except at the proximal splenic flexure where the folds are thickened and edematous. In M. G. this is undoubtedly submucosal hemorrhage caused by his fall. Radiographically the appearance and location are also compatible with ischemic colitis, which commonly occurs at the splenic flexure where the middle and left colic arteries anastomose.

Mr. M. G. is relieved at the findings on the barium enema. He is supposed to return to your office in one week for a follow-up visit, but he calls and says he is feeling fine and will not be in.

Barium examination is the simplest way to look for hemorrhage into the bowel wall. If perforation is a clinical consideration, water soluble contrast medium can be substituted. The radiographic findings are often non-specific and must be correlated with the clinical history.

J. H. is a 23 year old itinerant logger whose frequent job switching causes him trouble because he barely learns the local customs before he moves on. You see him after a logging truck has run over his abdomen. He had signalled it to go forward but instead, the driver, mistaking his sign, reversed. Though he initially did not seem badly hurt, the company helicopter was called to evacuate him to the county hospital where you examine him about five hours after the injury. By now he has fairly severe abdominal pain. His white cell count is elevated, and he has microscopic hematuria. First you order an excretory urogram. The preliminary film and a 10 minute film are shown. What do you see?

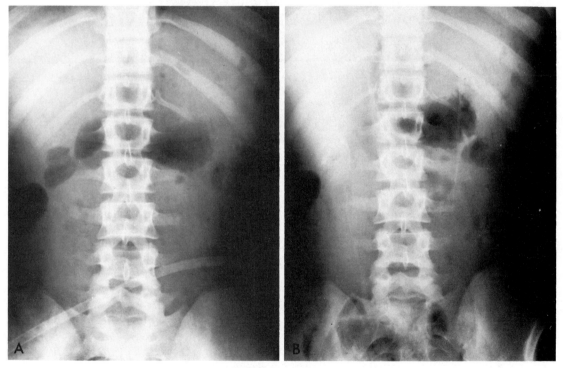

Figure 4–4a, b

The preliminary film shows a single, dilated loop of small bowel to the left of L1 that looks edematous. In addition, there are some bubbles of gas at about T11–T12 on the left that do not seem to be within bowel. Neither kidney nor psoas margin is seen. The 10 minute film demonstrates good renal excretion bilaterally. Using the entire excretory urogram, you conclude that the kidney contours are normal, as are the collecting systems and the ureters. The apparently extraluminal gas collections are still seen. What would you consider doing now?

Because of extraluminal gas, you consider laparotomy but decide to do an upper gastrointestinal series using water soluble contrast material first. At fluoroscopy you know you have hit pay dirt. What makes you so sure?

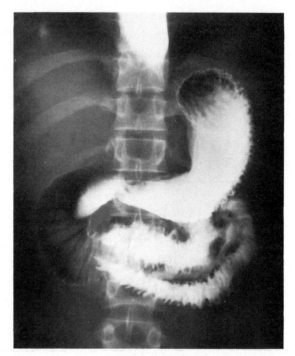

Figure 4–4c

The stomach is normal and the duodenum is somewhat distended. The proximal jejunum is edematous with irregular, thickened folds, and there is immediate extravasation of contrast material from the lumen. J. H. has a small bowel laceration requiring prompt resection and repair.

Bowel rupture caused by blunt trauma is not very common and can be difficult to diagnose unless it is clinically suspected. Delayed diagnosis will increase the morbidity of the injury. Isolated bowel injury may be asymptomatic early in its course, becoming apparent only when peritonitis or abscess occurs. Bowel rupture can also be masked by other abdominal injuries in the patient with severe trauma.

J. H. has a difficult postoperative course with a prolonged ileus and a subphrenic abscess. It will be months before he resumes logging, and you encourage him to find some other, safer, occupation.

MASTER R. B., J. M., MRS. M. B., MR. M. E. AND K. S.

The five patients included in this case illustrate the many approaches that may be available for a single diagnostic problem. The clinician and diagnostician must be aware of all such modalities and choose the ones that are most likely to be effective in a specific patient. Factors to be considered include the ability of patient to cooperate, speed with which the procedure can be accomplished, the risk to the patient, cost of the procedure and concomitant diagnostic problems, among others. This decision process should take very little time once you are aware of what each procedure entails.

Master R. B. is a typical eight year old, so when he arrives home in tears after falling off a swing his mother is not overly concerned. She does become concerned when he is still lying on his bed clutching his stomach half an hour later, and about one hour after his fall, she decides to bring R. B. to your office. R. B. tells you he was standing on the swing when he lost his footing and fell off, but you can't find out what part he fell on. Your physical examination, however, is rewarding. R. B. is quite tender in his left upper quadrant and will not let you palpate that area. The rest of his abdomen is soft. When you hear that his hemoglobin is 10.5 mg%, you are concerned about splenic injury with bleeding. You request supine and upright abdominal films and discuss with the radiologist the various procedures available to confirm your diagnosis.

The upight abdominal film is illustrated. What do you see?

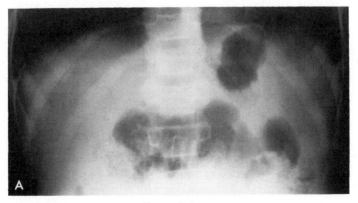

Figure 4–5a

Gas is present in the transverse colon and stomach. While the spleen cannot be precisely defined, the stomach is displaced medially, the splenic flexure is low and there is a soft tissue fullness in the left upper quadrant.

After further discussion with the radiologist you decide to order an isotopic spleen scan. R. B. is quite tender, and you think he will be unable to cooperate with the ultrasonographer, who will have to press the ultrasound transducer into his sore side, and he is wriggling too much for CT.

A film from the scan is demonstrated. What do you see?

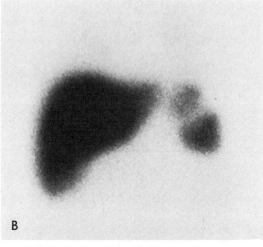

Figure 4–5b

The liver is normal on this anteroposterior scan. The spleen has an oblique cleft indicative of a laceration.

Diagnosis confirmed, the decision is made to attempt a partial splenectomy, since R. B. now has a rapid pulse rate and feels faint. The surgery is accomplished easily, and R. B. recuperates quickly.

J. M., an older woman who does not want to accept the limitations that sometimes come with age, falls from a ladder while painting the ceiling in her home. At first she is primarily concerned about the dreadful mess that the spilled paint caused. Later in the day, when she continues to be bothered by pain on her side and feels weak, she calls for an appointment. You decide to meet her at the hospital, since you know she tries to minimize her complaints.

Examination shows a large bruise on the left side, with marked tenderness in the left upper quadrant of the abdomen. She also complains of pain on deep breathing and has tachycardia. Your presumptive diagnosis is a splenic rupture, and you order an ultrasound examination.

The examination is difficult to perform because J. M. is in pain, though she tries to be stoic. There is also a large amount of bowel gas in the left abdomen. Finally, some good sections are obtained in the right lateral decubitus position. Do these confirm the diagnosis? Remember, the spleen is normally homogenous and rather echo-free.

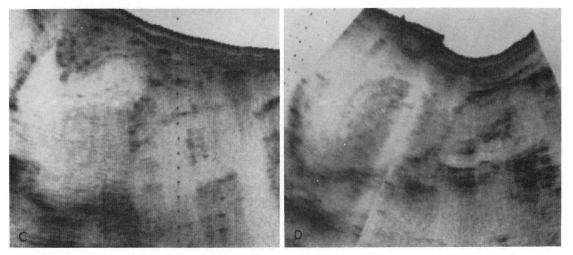

Figure 4-5c, d

The spleen, seen between the diaphragm and the left kidney, is enlarged, and in its inferomedial aspect there is a large, rounded area of echo-producing material. While these findings could be caused by any echogenic mass in the splenic hilum, the sonographer is confident that, in this context, it is a mass of clots. There is also a small amount of free fluid in the subhepatic space on sections not illustrated.

J. M. is taken promptly to surgery and the finding of splenic hematoma is confirmed. She does well without her spleen and soon is as feisty as ever.

Sonographic diagnosis of spleen trauma may be quite difficult because of a variety of factors, including inability of the patient to cooperate because of pain, position of the spleen high under the ribs, acoustical shadowing by gas and the variable and often subtle nature of the findings. It is important that multiple projections be tried before the examination is abandoned.

Mr. M. E. and Mrs. M. B. came to the emergency room nearly simultaneously because of blunt injuries to the left upper quadrant. Mr. M. E. hit his left side on a railing falling off a bar stool. His drinking companions initially ignored his complaints, but when a few more drinks did not get rid of the pain, they poured him into a car and brought him to the hospital. Mrs. M. B. was skiing in the Sierras when an out-of-control "hot-dogger" knocked her down. She had skied for another hour or so, but felt poorly and was driven down from the mountains to see you.

Both patients are tender in the left upper quadrant and both have bloody peritoneal lavages, though Mrs. M. B. has grossly bloody fluid while Mr. M. E. has only a pink-tinged return. Both are mildly anemic, and in each patient you are concerned about splenic injury. You again consider the several ways to evaluate splenic trauma. Mr. M. E. certainly will not hold still for an ultrasound of his spleen. The problem is compounded by the need for a really good inspiratory effort by the patient. You consider a CT, but Mr. M. E. is thrashing around so much that you decide to request celiac angiography. Preliminary film for the angiogram reveals many metallic fragments superimposed over the spleen. You remember picking buckshot out of Mr. M. E. a few years back when he attempted to rob a gas station.

Three films from the celiac injection are shown. They were taken at 1, 2.5 and 5 seconds after the start of the contrast medium injection. Does Mr. M. E. have significant splenic injury? What are the angiographic findings of splenic trauma?

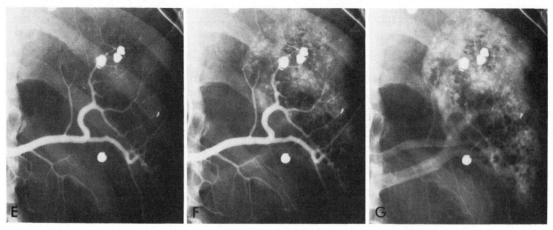

Figure 4–5e, f, g

The first film shows the buckshot that M. E. has had for some time. The splenic artery is normal. Pancreatic branches arise from its caudal surface. The intrasplenic arterial branches show slight irregularity in caliber, and there is some subtle stretching of arteries, especially in the upper pole. The second film is much more dramatic. There is very irregular mottled parenchymal accumulation of contrast material throughout most of the spleen and also early filling of the splenic vein. The final film shows dense filling of the splenic vein and again demonstrates the irregular parenchymal accumulation of contrast material. Splenic lacerations are seen as linear voids in the parenchymal phase. Mr. M. E. has at least three lacerations.

At surgery, there is little free blood in the abdomen. The spleen is swollen and discolored and of abnormal consistency. There is a small capsular laceration. When the spleen is taken out, it is bivalved and is seen to be markedly contused and fractured.

Other angiographic abnormalities that can be seen with splenic injury include frank extravasation of contrast material into a laceration, wedge-shaped defects in the parenchymal stain caused by hematomas, and subcapsular collections of blood, which stretch the capsular arteries and usually deform the splenic parenchyma into a crescentic shape, displacing the spleen from the body wall.

Though angiography is highly accurate in the evaluation of splenic injury, it provides more information than the surgeon usually needs. At the current time, most spleens with significant injury are removed and anatomical information is generally not needed. As partial splenectomy becomes more common in the young, however, angiography may again become more important. You are happy, therefore, that Mrs. M. B., though in pain, is able to cooperate for a CT scan. Ultrasound was not successful because her spleen was high up under her ribs and she just could not take in a deep enough breath.

Three scans from the CT are shown. They are all made after 300 cc of 25 per cent contrast medium was infused intravenously. The first two scans are 2 cm apart and the third 3 cm further caudad. What do you see?

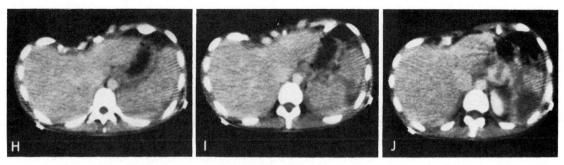

Figure 4–5h, i, j

The highest section shows an unusual configuration of the anterior abdominal wall caused by a childhood injury. The aorta and portal veins are faintly opacified with contrast material. The spleen is large but shows no intrinsic abnormalties on this section. There is a soft tissue collection dorsal to the spleen, which you think may be hemorrhage from the spleen. The next section shows a band of low attenuation extending from the splenic hilum through the spleen. Once again, there is an adjacent hematoma. The final section is just below the spleen and shows a mottled, irregular mass that is also probably blood. The upper pole of the left kidney is seen medially on this section.

Surgery confirms your interpretation of the CT scans, and Mrs. M. B. is anxious to go skiing before the season ends. Her convalescence is smooth, and six weeks after her injury you hear she has gone up to Tahoe for the corn snow.

As mentioned earlier, most severely injured spleens are removed shortly after diagnosis either because of the danger of delayed catastrophic hemorrhage or to control acute bleeding. A certain percentage of splenic injuries will be diagnosed clinically or will be found at laparotomy. In patients in whom there is a question of splenic trauma in a non-urgent clinical setting, a variety of radiographic studies can be used. Plain radiographs of the abdomen may show lower rib fractures or displacement of viscera adjacent to the spleen. These findings are not diagnostic but heighten concern. The absence of plain film abnormality certainly does not exclude splenic injury. The choice of further imaging modalities will depend upon the patient, local practice and availability. The isotopic spleen scan can provide useful information, but variations in anatomy can lead to false positive diagnoses. Ultrasound examination of the spleen is often difficult in the face of trauma and is highly dependent on operator patience and skill.

As we have seen in these exercises, CT scanning shows the spleen and adjacent organs well and will certainly show hematomas in and around the spleen. Splenic angiography is the most sensitive and specific examination available and will demonstrate splenic contusion without hematoma. It provides more detailed information, however, than is often needed unless it is important to save all or a portion of the spleen. In most circumstances ultrasound, CT or isotopic scanning will provide enough information for the clinician.

Even when you are fully aware of the diagnostic techniques best suited to make a certain diagnosis, it is possible to find yourself involved in a case in which the signs and symptoms are misleading and you reach the diagnosis through the back door. K. S. is such a patient.

K. S. is a 20 year old college student who spends as much time as possible in sporting activities. It is the season for both soccer and touch football, so you know he must feel awful to come to the school infirmary on a Saturday morning. He is a rather poor historian, but it seems that he feels weak and has no appetite. Over the last four days he has vomited once or twice and is nauseated most of the time.

When you examine him, you find several bruises that he cannot remember getting, but then he is always banged up. He has vague tenderness in the left upper quadrant also, but there are no palpable masses or organomegaly. Laboratory results are not helpful except that his hematocrit is 34 mg%, which is somewhat low for a young man. His white count is slightly elevated, but there is no left shift.

Mystified, but sure K. S. is ill, you talk to him at some length. The only meager clue seems to be stress and worry about his neglected academic studies. He is way behind, has several papers due and has been given "probable failure" notice in three courses. His father has threatened to withdraw his support unless K. S. does better. This makes you wonder if K. S. has a duodenal ulcer. Since he has not eaten breakfast, you request an upper gastrointestinal series for that morning and send him to radiology.

About half an hour later, the radiologist calls you. He has just seen the preliminary abdominal film for the upper gastrointestinal series. The film is illustrated, and there are two pertinent observations. Can you make them?

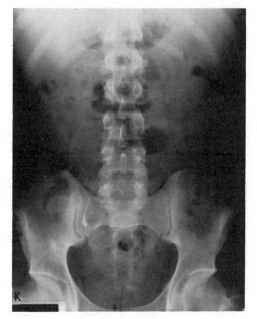

Figure 4-5k

The film, at first glance, may seem quite unremarkable and, to a large extent, it is. However, looking at the left upper quadrant, you should wonder about splenic enlargement. The splenic tip is below the costal margin and is bulbous. More significant is the presence of triangular soft tissue shadows above and lateral to the bladder, perhaps more obvious on the right. These are sometimes called "dog ears" and are a sign of intraperitoneal fluid. The radiologist asks if he should go ahead with the study and, still in a quandary, you agree. No ulcer is found, but the study does help to answer the question about the spleen. A single film from the gastrointestinal series is illustrated on the following page. What do you think?

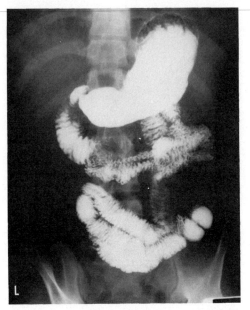

Figure 4–51

The spleen is definitely enlarged and is displacing both stomach and small bowel. Splenic injury with bleeding should have come to mind somewhere during this tale, but K. S. cannot remember any specific injury, and his left upper quadrant is free of bruises. You perform a four quadrant abdominal tap and get back bloody fluid on the first needling. One of the consulting surgeons for the college is passing the examining room, so you call him in to see K. S. The surgeon recognizes K. S. and asks how he is doing after being rammed in the side at the football game four days ago. The impact had momentarily stunned K. S. but obviously had made a greater impression on the watching surgeon than on K. S.

K. S. is more than reluctant when you tell him he needs to have his spleen removed. Even the surgeon cannot convince him of the need for an operation. When his girlfriend arrives, you explain the dilemma to her and she gets K. S. to agree to hospitalization and observation. His hematocrit continues to drop slowly but continually, and his spleen becomes clearly palpable over the next two days. Faced with this, he agrees to splenectomy.

At operation about 300 cc of bloody intraperitoneal fluid is found. The spleen is large, discolored and tense. When it is removed, a large subcapsular hematoma is found. There is only a rather small parenchymal laceration.

K. S. illustrates one of the problems that can be encountered with splenic injury. The symptoms and signs can be quite nonspecific, and without a clear-cut history of trauma, the diagnosis may not be initially considered. He also underlines the fact that there are many ways to reach the diagnosis of splenic injury, though this particular path would not be the one of choice.

MRS. S., A. A., MS. M. B. AND J. J.

The four patients in this case illustrate some of the problems inherent in liver trauma. The liver is a large solid organ that becomes harder with age. In the young, deep stellate lacerations can occur which are not palpable at surgery, while in the adult, lacerations are more likely to reach the surface of the liver. Subcapsular hematomas occur as well as capsular lacerations which may be associated with serious hemorrhage. Liver injury may not be apparent immediately after an injury but may become symptomatic days to weeks later, presenting with pain or jaundice or hemobilia.

Many hepatic injuries require no surgical intervention, since they will heal with conservative therapy. In those cases that need surgery, the surgeon may want a "roadmap" such as is provided by angiography to accurately identify the injured hepatic segment. In other situations, CT or ultrasound will be sufficient. The patients who are illustrated demonstrate acute and delayed problems caused by hepatic injury.

The irrepressible Mrs. S. has just called about another of her misadventures. It seems she was rock climbing at Yosemite over the weekend and had a "slight" fall. This is both remarkable and alarming in a woman of 71, and you ask her to meet you at the emergency room.

On examination, she has some scrapes on both calves and is quite tender over the right lower rib cage. Rib radiographs do not show any fractures, and you are about to send her home when you are told that her hematocrit is 31 mg%, her bilirubin 2.1 mg%, and her SGOT 150 mU/ml with an LDH of 247 mU/ml. You suspect liver injury and insist on hospitalization and an emergency liver scan. The AP and posterior oblique views of a ^{99}Tc sulfur colloid liver scan are shown on the following page. What do you see?

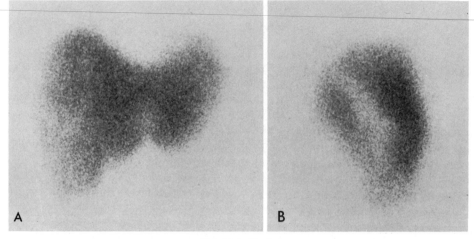

Figure 4–6a, b

There is an extensive defect in the colloid uptake in the right lobe. The oblique view shows a prominent linear component to the defect. This is compatible with an extensive liver injury, and a CT scan is recommended to more fully define the injury. The section illustrated is performed following infusion of intravenous contrast. What do you think?

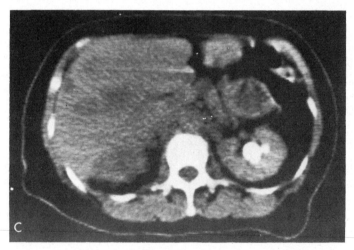

Figure 4–6c

There is an irregular band-like area of diminished attenuation extending transversely across the right lobe that is compatible with a laceration, though no hematoma is identified. You discuss Mrs. S. with the surgeon, who feels that close observation is appropriate and that surgery can probably be avoided. She requests hepatic angiography to define the vascular anatomy in case urgent surgery is needed. What do you see on this celiac angiogram?

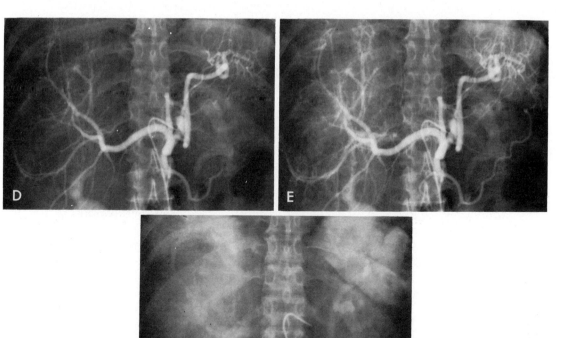

Figure 4–6d, e, f

On the early arterial film, there is splaying of the larger arteries in the mid-right lobe, which corresponds to the area of abnormality seen on the other two studies. Did you notice the small, rounded collection of contrast medium superimposed on the right tenth rib? This is a small pseudoaneurysm. There is filling of adjacent portal venous branches. The next film shows diffuse arterial-portal vein shunting, not only from the area of the pseudoaneurysm but from the entire injured area. The last film shows a large, irregularly marginated defect in the hepatogram.

Mrs. S. feels well and soon is clamoring to get up. She drives the nurses to distraction and is discharged five days later without further incident.

Hepatic laceration may be seen in a variety of presentations from life-threatening hemorrhage to delayed symptomatology following minimal trauma. The diagnostic approach must be tailored to the individual patient. As is seen in Mrs. S., several imaging techniques can be used to shed varying degrees of light on liver injury.

A. A. is an athletic, 68 year old woman who also doesn't quite accept her age. A year ago she had a comminuted fracture of her right leg, developed thrombophlebitis and then pulmonary emboli. She has been anticoagulated ever since. You are called into the emergency room to see her one Sunday evening because she is having severe upper abdominal pain and has fainted. It seems she went roller skating in Golden Gate Park in the early afternoon and was bowled over by a child on a skateboard. She struck her right side on the curb when she fell, but went on skating for another 20 or 30 minutes until she began to feel poorly. She went home but became increasingly uncomfortable and so caught a cab to the hospital.

She appears pale and her pulse is fast and thready when you see her. You sit her up and she again becomes faint. Her abdomen is swollen and tender. You cannot feel her liver edge, but can percuss it well below the costal margin — a marked enlargement from recent examinations. You draw blood for hemoglobin, hematocrit and possible crossmatching and arrange for an emergency CT scan of the upper abdomen. What is your working diagnosis?

Three sections from the CT scan are shown. A. A. has been given some dilute oral contrast material, which is still in her stomach. No intravenous contrast material has been given. Can you confirm your diagnosis?

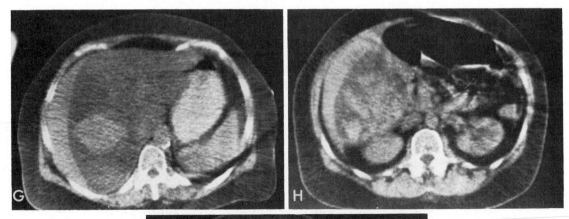

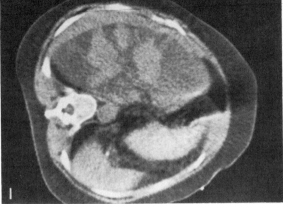

Figure 4–6g, h, i

The first two sections are done with the patient in the supine position, while the third is performed with A. A. in a left lateral decubitus position. Why might her position have been changed?

The observations to be made are common to all three sections. The CT attenuation of the liver is less than that of the spleen or kidneys, which is unusual. There is a crescentic area of higher attenuation lateral to the liver and several irregular but rather ovoid areas of higher attenuation within the liver substance. You feel sure that your working diagnosis of hepatic injury with bleeding is confirmed. There are both subcapsular and intraparenchymal hemorrhages. The radiologist agrees and also explains that A. A. was placed in the decubitus position to decrease respiratory motion. Breath holding was quite painful for her and she was unable to do so after the first few sections.

You admit A. A. and transfuse her. She must have bled massively, since she needs nine units of blood to stabilize her hematocrit at about 40 mg%. Though her prothrombin time was not excessively low when she was admitted, you decide not to maintain her on anticoagulation.

About 10 weeks after this incident, you see A. A. again. She obviously has hepatitis, which distresses, but doesn't overly surprise you. To be sure that her hepatic subcapsular hematoma is not compressing hepatic tissue, you obtain a repeat CT scan. What do you see now?

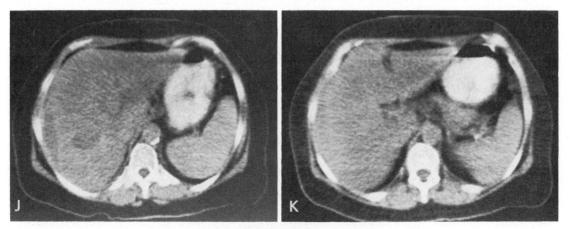

Figure 4–6j, k

The crescentic subcapsular collection is still seen but is now of lower attenuation than the liver. The areas of hemorrhage are much smaller in volume, and you feel that she is resorbing the multiple areas of hemorrhage.

CT provides a simple way to evaluate the liver for hemorrhage. When surgical intervention is not planned, it is usually the procedure of choice, though both ultrasound and isotope scans can be used. Angiography gives more detailed information and will often be requested when surgery is contemplated.

Ms. M. B. took up karate for self-defense and you suspect she is not getting proper training, since she has had a series of injuries in the past few months. When you see her this time, she has pain in the right upper quadrant and a sensation of fullness. You find out that she was kicked so hard in the right ribs about three weeks ago that she has not been back to her karate class. On examination, she is tender over the lower-right ribs, and it is difficult to examine her abdomen because of guarding but you think her liver is enlarged. When the laboratory reports moderately abnormal liver function tests and a hematocrit of 30 mg%, you request an ultrasound of the abdomen with attention to the liver.

What considerations have made you request an ultrasound? As you go to the ultrasound suite, you think about the vagaries of hepatic trauma. Unless the trauma is very severe, these injuries can remain occult for weeks before causing pain or jaundice or hemobilia. Late findings of trauma include subcapsular hematomas as well as intrahepatic collections. You wonder if there is a bleeding pseudoaneurysm and if angiography will be necessary.

The ultrasonographer is excited about his findings. One transverse scan done about 5 cm below the xyphoid and two longitudinal scans made 3 cm and 7 cm to the right of midline are demonstrated. What do you see?

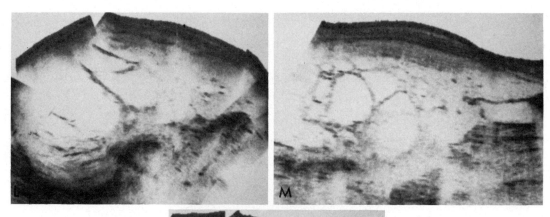

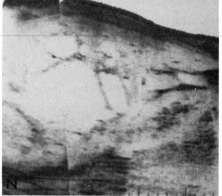

Figure 4–6l, m, n

All three scans show transonic masses within the enlarged liver. Though the masses are transonic like fluid, there is no enhanced transmission through them, suggesting that they are not simple cysts. With the history Ms. M. B. gives, organized hematomas seem most likely.

Initially, you plan conservative therapy but Ms. M. B. has increasing abdominal distress and requires surgery. You diagnosis is confirmed. Before discharge you try to convince her that age 55 is not a good time to take a course in martial arts.

⚜

You fully expect to find J. J. up and about when you make morning rounds. He is now seven days post right hepatectomy for liver trauma caused by a car versus tree crash at about 40 miles an hour. At 18, he should bounce back. Instead, he is lying in bed looking yellowish-gray and feeling awful. On examination, he is distinctly jaundiced and feels warm. His abdomen, however, is not unduly tender and you feel no masses.

Chart review does not ease your mind. J. J. has run a low-grade fever ever since surgery. It should be regressing but you see that the trend is up and he has hit 39°C in the last 24 hours. His bilirubin, which rose as expected after surgery, has continued to rise. It should be falling. The white cell count remains elevated, and there is an increasing shift to the left.

You review in your mind the night of J. J.'s admission. Four seriously injured teenagers were brought in from the crash. The car had apparently gone off the road on a curve at about 40 mph, hit a large tree, sending one rider through the windshield, and then turned over at least twice, ending upside down. Two of the boys were unresponsive, one from a head injury and J. J. from shock, when they arrived in the emergency room. J. J. had been rushed to surgery when a needle placed into his abdomen produced a spurt of bright red blood. The large amount of blood seen on entering the abdomen could not obscure an extensive liver laceration in the right lobe. Gaining control of the bleeding was very difficult, and 16 units of blood were given during surgery and several more were required in the next 24 hours. After removing the lacerated right lobe, a T-tube was placed and drains were left in place. When the operation was complete, you were more concerned about possible complications secondary to shock rather than hepatic problems. The former have not occurred, but now you are facing the latter. As you leaf through the chart, the surgical pathology report catches your eye. The first sentence reads in part, "A rather small, badly lacerated right hepatic lobe," and you are sure what the problem is. The resection was not really a total right hepatectomy. The right hepatic artery was ligated and the right portal vein was tied off, but there was residual right hepatic tissue, not an uncommon occurrence at emergency partial hepatectomy. The devascularized segment is producing the jaundice, the fever and the elevated white count. At this point supportive care would probably suffice, but you wish to confirm your impression, so you request a hepatic angiogram.

The celiac angiogram is performed later that day. Two films taken at three and 15 seconds after the start of the contrast medium injection are shown. What do you see?

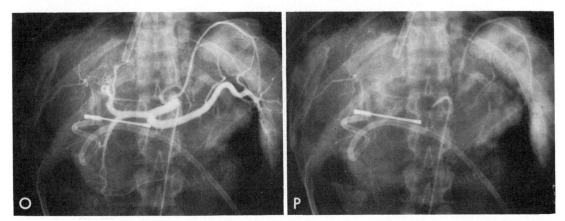

Figure 4–6o, p

The stump of the right hepatic artery is seen near the cephalad limb of the T-tube. The left hepatic arterial branches are larger than usual, as would be expected in a regenerating liver. There are right hepatic arteries supplied by collateral arteries from the left hepatic arterial distribution, a common collateral pathway. On the second film at 15 seconds these right hepatic arteries are still filled, indicating how poor the circulation is in this segment of the liver. The splenic vein is already opacified.

With the cause of his prolonged convalescence clear, J. J. begins to improve and goes home about seven days later. You hope he does not get hepatitis from his transfusions. All goes well until about two days before the day set to remove J. J.'s T-tube. Once again, you are the senior surgeon for the emergency room and once again a car of teenagers has crashed, this time into some parked cars. J. J. is the least hurt. He does have a mildly positive peritoneal lavage for blood, however. It is now six weeks since the first crash and five since the angiogram. You doubt anything is seriously wrong with J. J., but you can feel his spleen. Rather than observe J. J. you decide to order a repeat angiogram to exclude significant splenic or other injury. The angiogram shows no evidence of acute injury, but it is interesting to compare it to the previous angiogram. What do you see on the film?

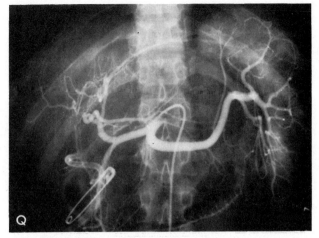

Figure 4–6q

First, the spleen is larger. This is a normal response to partial hepatectomy and occurs because of both portal hypertension and a proliferation of the reticuloendothelial cells in the spleen. Second, the left hepatic arterial branches are larger and are much farther apart. This is caused by hepatic regeneration. Finally, there has been an increase in the collateral arteries to the residual right lobe.

J. J.'s T-tube is accidentally removed with the sterile drapes following the angiogram. He doesn't turn a hair and leaves the hospital the following day. You suggest he find friends who are better drivers! J. J. thinks that is a reasonable idea, but the next time you hear of him he has taken up bobsledding. This time he is the driver.

F. T.

F. T. comes to your office with abdominal pain, nausea and vomiting. When you examine him, you are sure there is an abdominal mass. On close questioning, he dates the onset of pain to a Saturday morning "pickup" football game in which he found himself repeatedly at the bottom of a heap of tacklers. After placing a nasogastric tube, you decide to get a plain film of the abdomen. What do you see?

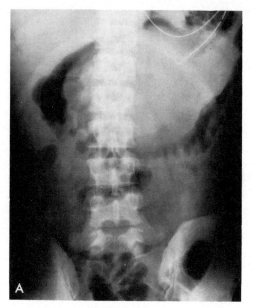

Figure 4–7a

There is a large mass in the upper abdomen, displacing the stomach cephalad and the transverse colon caudad. The duodenal sweep is dilated and widened. These findings all suggest a pancreatic mass. In view of the history, traumatic pancreatitis with development of a pseudocyst is likely, although other causes, such as a hematoma, an abscess or a neoplasm, must be considered.

You order an abdominal ultrasound. Selected transverse and longitudinal sections are illustrated. What do you make of them?

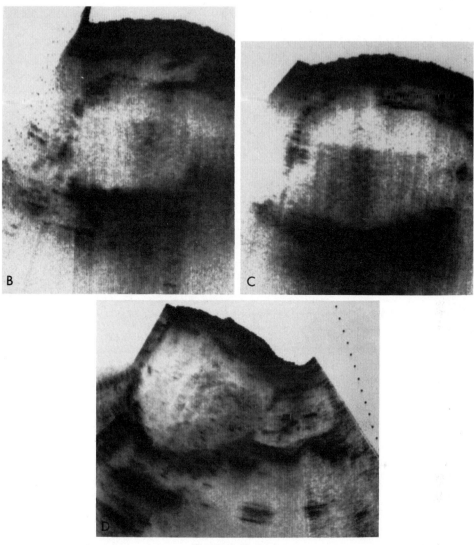

Figure 4–7b, c, d

There is a large ovoid mass in the mid abdomen. It is relatively transonic, but in the dependent part of the mass there is echogenic material. The appearance is compatible with a pseudocyst of the pancreas, though a hematoma or abscess could look like this. The presence of an elevated amylase reinforces the diagnosis of pseudocyst. At surgery, some time later, a large pancreatic pseudocyst with internal debris is found and is marsupialized to the stomach.

Traumatic pancreatic pseudocysts are uncommon. They are most frequent in children and adolescents, since the costal arch is still pliable and can compress the pancreas against the spine, disrupting the pancreatic ductal system. The formation of the pseudocyst follows pancreatic necrosis and exudation of fluid. Radiologic techniques used to demonstrate traumatic pseudocysts are no different from those used for their non-traumatic brethren. CT and ultrasound are the simplest and most informative techniques. Endoscopic retrograde pancreatography will show the relationship of the cyst to the duct system but is sometimes difficult and may lead to infection of the pseudocyst. Other injuries to the pancreas, such as laceration, generally accompany very severe abdominal injuries. If the patient survives the initial trauma, radiologic techniques, including CT, ultrasound and even angiography, often have a role in the convalescent period.

C. S.

There is little to be said about C. S. She is a chronic uncontrolled schizophrenic who has been institutionalized for 16 of her 30 years. She spends much time and effort on escape attempts, and one technique she has used repeatedly is serious self-injury requiring hospitalization. This time she has swallowed several long, sharp objects and is sent over for evaluation and whatever care is needed. The attendant who brings C. S. in has AP and lateral abdominal films with him. What do you see?

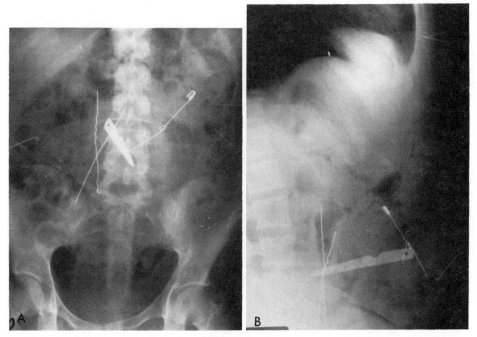

Figure 4–8a, b

You sigh as you look at the films because it seems unlikely that you can avoid operating once again on C. S. Open hair pins, one open large safety pin and a nail file are all seen in the abdominal cavity. With these two views it seems unlikely that all are completely intraluminal at this time and, even if they are, you cannot imagine safe passage of all of these items. The other metallic foreign bodies are old, and you know they are in soft tissue. There are two needles in her left breast seen on the lateral film and another needle in her left flank. A piece of a paper clip is in her abdominal wall on the right. Metallic sutures are also seen.

At surgery, all four new foreign bodies had perforated the bowel. The nail file and one hair pin were entirely in the peritoneal cavity while the other two were still partly in bowel. Adhesions from previous surgery complicated this operation but also probably decreased spillage from the new holes. All in all, C. S. does well but you dread her next return.

As you have seen in earlier cases, radiology is important in localization of foreign bodies. When the foreign bodies are radiopaque, plain films will often be sufficient. In this case, a small bowel series was considered but not performed, since surgery was necessary regardless of the position of the foreign bodies. In other situations, contrast studies will be useful. As in so much of trauma radiology, the examination needs to be planned for the specific patient, since each of these problems is unique.

MS. S. M. AND MS. V. Y.

S. M. is a 19 year old who has recently moved into an apartment that she is sharing with her boyfriend. Neither one is particularly organized and so things do go wrong. This time S. M. has taken a large drink out of a beer bottle by her work stand and has had immediate burning chest pain. It turns out that the bottle contained a concentrated lye solution that her boyfriend was planning to use to make soap. He rushes her to the emergency room where you order an esophagram. What do you see on this film of the esophagus?

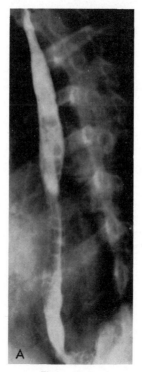

Figure 4-9a

The esophagus is narrowed just below the crossing of the left mainstem bronchus. The wall of the esophagus is thickened. The picture may look rather benign, but the fibrosis that occurs in such chemical injuries can lead to severe strictures. S. M. does have increasing trouble swallowing over the next few weeks, and six weeks later you order a repeat esophagram, which is shown on the following page. What has happened?

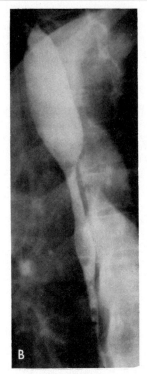

Figure 4–9b

The proximal esophagus is now quite dilated, and there is a significant stenosis of the mid esophagus with loss of mucosal detail. It is difficult to know how long the stricture is because there is no way to distend the esophagus below the lesion.

S. M. does not respond to conservative treatment, and dilation is not effective. About six months after her acid ingestion, she has to have a colon interposition type procedure to bypass the stricture. This goes well, but you fear she will have more disasters over the years.

Despondent over an unhappy love life, V. Y. drinks concentrated acid. Unbelievable searing pain and vomiting bring her to the emergency room where supportive measures are instituted along with treatment with antacids. After a few days you order an upper GI. Here is a view of the stomach and duodenum. What are the findings?

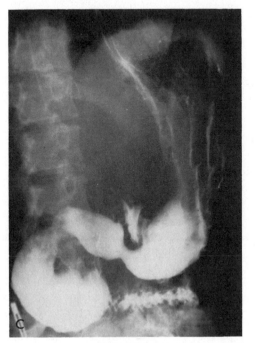

Figure 4–9c

The mucosal folds in the body of the stomach are markedly thickened and shaggy. There is effacement of the mucosal pattern in the antrum and duodenum with dilation of the duodenum. There has obviously been an extensive mucosal and submucosal acid injury to all these areas.

After a prolonged hospitalization for her medical and psychological problems, V. Y. is ready for discharge. A follow-up gastrointestinal series is shown on the following page. What do you see now?

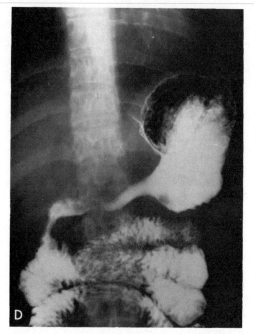

Figure 4–9d

There is now narrowing of the antrum, duodenal bulb and descending duodenum. This stricturing is due to fibrosis occurring in the healing process and was expected. You fear that the process may go on to obstruction, but V. Y. is anxious to leave the hospital. Ultimately, she does return because of abdominal pain and vomiting and requires surgery to relieve the obstruction.

Ingestion of strong acid solutions is more likely to damage the stomach and duodenum than the esophagus, the reverse of alkali ingestion, though large volumes and concentrated solutions may damage all parts of the upper gastrointestinal tract. Radiologic evaluation is important in assessing extent of injury and is invaluable for following the healing process.

CHAPTER
5

GENITOURINARY TRACT

INTRODUCTION

Since the pancreas has been included in the chapter on gastrointestinal trauma, most of the remaining trauma to the retroperitoneum involves the genitourinary tract. The kidneys are the most frequently injured portion of this system, but injuries to the ureters, bladder and urethra often present more serious management problems. Injuries to the pregnant uterus are rarely radiologic problems but can have important clinical implications. Injuries to the non-pregnant uterus are uncommon but may also present difficult diagnostic dilemmas. Severe soft tissue injuries to the pelvis are usually associated with multiple fractures of the pelvic ring, which often distract clinical attention from the concomitant soft tissue injuries. However, urethral disruption and bladder laceration occur with these fractures and must be identified. Injuries to branches of the internal iliac artery are also a frequent companion of severe pelvic fractures. These may lead to serious hemorrhage and are best found by angiography and treated with angiographic embolization in most circumstances.

Penetrating injuries often involve the retroperitoneum either with or without involvement of the abdomen. Need for radiology either at the time of injury or in the convalescent period is usually limited, though there are exceptions to this, especially if major vascular trauma is suspected. Knowledge of the variety of studies available for use in retroperitoneal injury is important so that the appropriate examinations can be used in a logical sequence.

CASE 5–1:

S. T., MASTER J. N., J. H. AND S. G.

S. T. turned his back on a man who was trying to bait him into a barroom fight. This gentlemanly act earned him a sharp kick in the right loin which sent him sprawling, and only the immediate arrival of the police spared him further blows. When he comes to the emergency room, his major complaint is right-sided, colicky pain, and a urinary catheter produces bloody urine. An intravenous urogram is requested. What does it show?

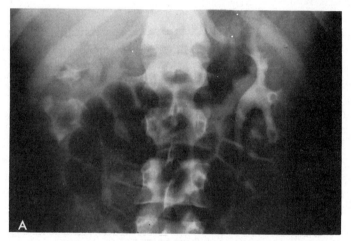

Figure 5–1a

This "cross kidney" view shows a marked difference in the two kidneys. The renal outlines, while hard to see, are intact and normal bilaterally. The right renal pelvis is distorted and has a large filling defect, which is probably a large thrombus. There is no renal displacement.

Since S. T. is clinically stable and both kidneys are excreting contrast material, further evaluation at this time is not felt to be indicated. He is admitted to the urology service for observation and does well. His urine clears slowly, and a repeat urogram two weeks later is normal.

Bleeding into the renal pelvis due to disruption of small blood vessels is not uncommon in blunt renal trauma. This bleeding is usually self-limited and usually does not require further evaluation or therapy unless there is obstruction or continued bleeding.

The late afternoon quiet of your office is shattered by the abrupt and unexpected arrival of Master J. N. and his highly agitated parents. J. N. has been your patient for his entire six years and you can tell from a distance that he is really in pain. To complicate matters, his shy, retiring mother is in tears and his father is demanding immediate attention but will not put J. N. down on your examining table. It takes an emphatic order to get J. N.'s parents to calm down. Once they do, his father tells you that the family had gone for an early afternoon walk. They stopped for ice cream cones, which they ate sitting on a park bench. After finishing his cone, J. N. tried some gymnastics on the bench, but lost his balance and fell off, landing on his back on the concrete pavement. He began to cry immediately and refused to be touched. His parents did not believe he could be really hurt, but he would not stop crying so they carried him home, becoming increasingly concerned about the possibility of a serious injury. When there was blood in his urine, they rushed hysterically to your office.

J. N. is still wailing and when you approach him, he begins to cry even more. He will not let you touch his right side, though you may carefully examine his left abdomen and listen to his chest. He really does not want to move at all and keeps sobbing that he hurts. When you confirm the presence of blood in his urine, you are rather sure what has happened. What radiographic examination would you order at this juncture?

The nature of the injury, along with bloody urine, once again makes a renal injury a real possibility, so you request an intravenous urogram. The first film demonstrated is the preliminary film for this study. What do you see?

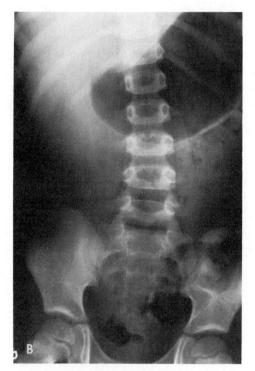

Figure 5–1b

There is a mild scoliosis of the lumbar spine with the convexity to the left consistent with the right-sided pain. No rib fractures are seen. While the left psoas margin and kidney are well seen, neither is visible on the right and, in fact, the entire right side of the abdomen is rather gray and gasless. You wonder about a large soft tissue mass below the liver. The next film is a 10 minute film from the urogram. What does it show?

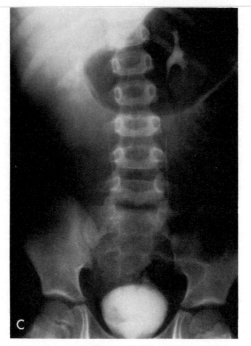

Figure 5–1c

The left kidney is normal. The collecting system is well seen, and the ureter is also normal. On the right, the collecting structures are ill-defined and distorted, and the renal contour is still not seen. There is some excretion, however, and the ureter is seen in part and is normal. You know at this point that J. N. has injured his right kidney and that it still has arterial supply and some function. Laboratory data reveal he has bled enough to drop his hemoglobin from 12 gm% on a recent examination to 10.2 gm% now, but his vital signs are stable, so, after consultation with a urologist, you decide to observe J. N., hoping to salvage his kidney.

All goes well for about 36 hours, but then J. N. complains of more pain and passes frank clots in his urine. His hemoglobin has dropped further, and when his pulse begins to go up, you order a follow-up urogram. What do you see on this coned-down, 10 minute film of the right kidney?

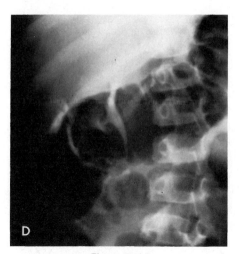

Figure 5-1d

The right kidney still functions, but now there is frank extravasation of contrast material beyond the collecting system lateral to the mid portion of the kidney. Because of continued evidence of bleeding from a renal laceration, you and the urologist feel J. N. must have surgical exploration and possible nephrectomy. You explain the situation to his parents, who consent. At surgery, the right kidney is found to have a fracture extending from the renal hilum through the parenchyma between the middle and lower third. There is a large perirenal hematoma. As feared, a partial nephrectomy is necessary but, as expected, J. N. bounces back, as children usually do, and is ready to go home in no time.

The intravenous urogram provides significant morphologic and physiologic information about the kidneys. This examination will usually be sufficient to diagnose the spectrum of renal trauma from contusion to gross rupture. Subcapsular and perirenal hematomas can usually be recognized because of compression or distortion of the nephrogram. There are certain situations where further studies, including ultrasound, CT and especially angiography, may be needed to further characterize the trauma. CT and ultrasound are particularly useful in defining the extent of hematomas. The patient who has sustained renal trauma and has non-visualization of the kidney at urography should generally have urgent angiography to evaluate the integrity of the renal vascular pedicle to separate severe contusion of the kidney from avulsion or thrombosis of the renal vessels, which require surgical intervention if the kidney is to be saved. Angiography may also be useful in the patient with uncontrolled post-traumatic hematuria when a partial nephrectomy is considered. The vascular anatomy is of importance to the surgeon in this situation. The patient with injury to a known solitary kidney should generally have early angiography in the face of the abnormal urogram, since detailed information is needed in these patients to help preserve as much renal tissue as possible.

Shortly after Master J. N. goes home, J. H. comes in, and she serves as a good example of some of these points.

Miss J. H. is very specific about her injury when she arrives at your office. Her horse kicked her in the left flank while she was grooming him for a show. Her side hurts and she has blood in her urine. After a quick examination, you order an emergency intravenous urogram; it shows a normal right kidney, a fractured left eleventh rib and no left renal function. The left psoas margin is not seen and there is a grayness to the left abdomen. You cannot see the left renal outline.

You admit Miss J. H., making her miss the horse show, and observe her vital signs and hematuria over the next day. When her hematocrit drops and her hematuria persists unabated, you request a left renal angiogram because surgery is now likely. Two arterial phase films are illustrated. What are your observations?

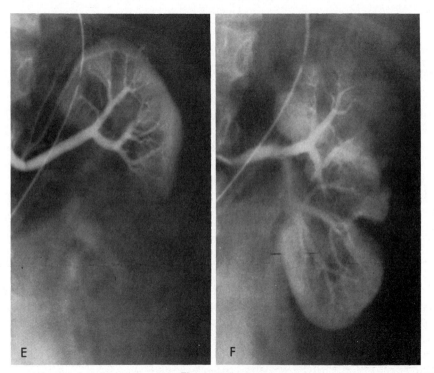

Figure 5–1e, f

Your first observation should be that there are at least two left renal arteries which arise from the aorta quite close to each other at the level of L1. The cephalad artery supplies a portion of the upper pole, which appears normal. The second renal artery supplies the remainder of the kidney, and you feel secure that the entire arterial supply to the kidney has been studied. If doubt persists, an aortogram could be performed. The injection of the second renal artery demonstrates several abnormalities. The first branch of this artery fills very poorly and has an unusual proximal course. The next branch fills better but tapers rapidly and ends abruptly. Several of its branches are amputated. The parenchymal accumulation of contrast material is abnormal. There are at least two linear defects across the mid portion of the kidney extending into the renal pelvis. Finally, you should wonder about extravasation of contrast material and blood caudad to the kidney. Without a preliminary film for comparison, this may be a difficult observation to confirm, but certainly the question should be raised on the films you have.

The angiographic findings in J. H. are typical of renal laceration with arterial disruption and parenchymal defects. Not infrequently, two renal arteries are found in patients with serious renal injury, perhaps because the double arterial supply makes the kidney less freely movable than in those with a single arterial supply. At least 20 per cent of kidneys have more than one major artery.

Miss J. H. agrees to surgical removal of her left kidney, which you recommend in light of her continued bleeding. Complete nephrectomy is necessary, but she recovers nicely and is back showing horses within the month.

⁓⁓

Unfortunately, or perhaps fortunately, not all renal trauma is so straightforward. The history may not be helpful and radiographs may be misleading or confusing. S. G. is such a patient.

S. G. is a 27 year old social butterfly who likes high-risk sports. Most recently, he has taken up hang gliding and skydiving and has had some rough landings. He arrives in your office looking quite pale and complains of severe left flank pain. Though he has no hematuria and the pain is not really typical of a kidney stone, you order an excretory urogram, since the problem seems to be renal in origin. A 10 minute film and a single tomographic section done after the 10 minute film are demonstrated. What do you see?

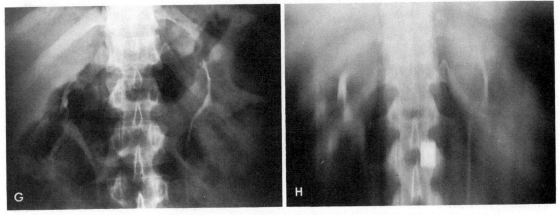

Figure 5–1g, h

The first observation you may make is that the left collecting system is spidery and effaced and that the lower pole calyces are not seen. The left renal contour is notable only for a shallow depression on the lateral surface seen best on the tomographic section. The right kidney is normal. Your tentative diagnosis of a renal stone seems unlikely, since a symptomatic renal stone causes dilatation of the calyces. Infection can lead to a spastic collecting system and masses can cause effacement, but there is little on the urogram, or in the clinical presentation, to support either diagnosis.

You admit S. G. to the hospital unsure of what is wrong. The only abnormality in his laboratory work is a hematocrit of 38%. His pain does not decrease over the next day, and a urologic consultant raises the possibility of exploratory surgery. Neither you nor S. G. find this idea at all appealing. You consider repeating the urogram, but the radiologist suggests a CT scan instead to look at the perirenal area in addition to evaluating the kidney with a different modality.

Four sections from the CT scan are demonstrated. The patient has been given dilute oral contrast material. The first two sections are done before intravenous contrast material is given and the last two, after. What observations can you make on these scans? Can you explain the urographic findings, and do you have a diagnosis?

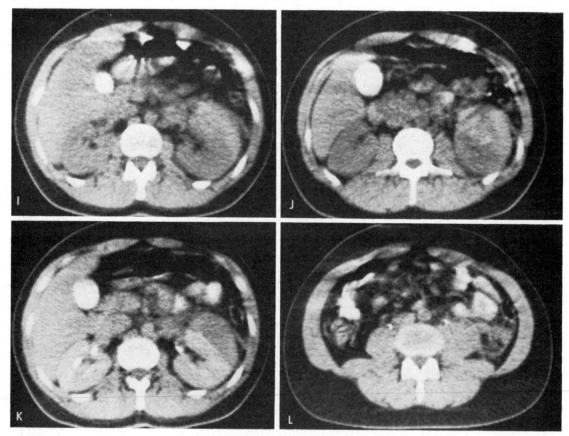

Figure 5–1i, j, k, l

The first two sections show that the left kidney is much larger than the right, which was not obvious on the urogram. More interesting is the crescentic area of higher attenuation on the ventral surface of the left kidney. What do you make of this? This collection should remind you of the hepatic subcapsular hematoma you saw earlier in this book and might even remind you of an acute subdural hematoma. An acute subcapsular hematoma of the kidney could cause S. G.'s symptoms and the findings on his urogram. The next section, made following the injection of intravenous contrast material, is at about the same level as Figure 5–1i. The kidney enhances, but the subcapsular collection does not. Contrast material would not readily enter a subcapsular hematoma. The last section, which is caudad to the kidneys, is quite interesting. There is blood in the perirenal space and along the left psoas muscle.

You are relieved to have an explanation of S. G.'s pain but now face the question of how or why he developed a subcapsular hematoma. Though S. G. pursues dangerous sports and would be unlikely to remember minor bumps and bruises, both he and several friends cannot remember any recent serious injury. He has no evidence of bleeding diathesis. When the question of a vasculitis or renal tumor as a bleeding cause is raised, you decide to request a renal angiogram to look for aneurysms or any other source of bleeding.

Three films from a selective left renal angiogram are demonstrated. They were taken at one, 2.5 and 4.5 seconds after the start of the contrast medium injection. What do you see?

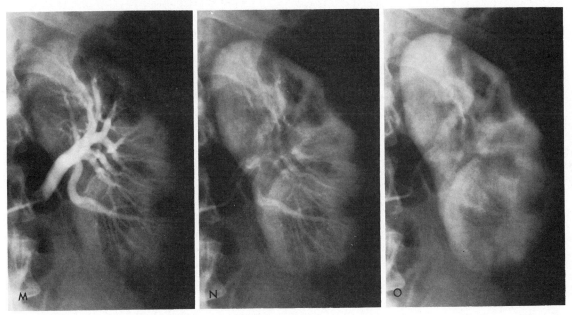

Figure 5–1m, n, o

The arteries to the kidney are large and they taper rather abruptly. This is a non-specific finding sometimes seen in hypertension. When you look at the smaller arteries on the one and 2.5 second films you see some fine irregularities in vessel caliber and also several punctate collections of contrast material, which should raise the question of small aneurysms. These are most apparent in the lower pole. On this injection, one of these collections persists into the early venous phase, good evidence for an aneurysm. A second projection is necessary to exclude the possibility of arteries seen on end. When this was done, at least five small aneurysms could be confirmed. Another observation is the indistinctness and irregularity of the lateral border of the kidney and the apparent separation of a lower pole capsular branch well away from the kidney itself. This latter finding is somewhat unreliable, since capsular arteries may not follow the renal contour exactly, but in this instance the capsular artery appears stretched. Steep oblique angiographic runs were performed in S. G. but did not add any more information.

The etiology of S. G.'s hematoma is still not certain, but there are at least three possible causes. The first is polyarteritis nodosa. Such patients bleed spontaneously and bleeding may be the first manifestation of the disease. S. G. has none of the other clinical manifestations of a systemic vasculitis, so this is felt to be unlikely. The second is a drug-induced necrotizing angiitis, which has an identical angiographic picture, but S. G. has not used drugs. Most probable in S. G. is simple trauma. Relatively non-specific trauma, such as occurs during a football game, can cause formation of small, generally transient pseudoaneurysms that may bleed either into the renal parenchyma or around it.

The decision is made to treat S. G. conservatively because his pain is receding. The major delayed problem of a renal subcapsular hematoma is development of a Page kidney from perirenal fibrosis. Mr. S. G. has no further trouble and follow-up urograms at six and 12 months are normal. He escapes without developing hypertension, and about 18 months later you hear he has gone to climb Mt. Everest.

V. S., P. R., MR. C. W. AND W. E.

V. S. is sent to see you because of increasing renal failure at age 27. As a child he was repeatedly ill and actually was tutored at home for both the third and fourth grades. His internist has been worrying about renal failure for several years and has an extensive record documenting a rising BUN and creatinine. V. S. is becoming symptomatic, and the latest urogram demonstrated virtually no function in small kidneys. Decisions now must be made about long-term dialysis and possible renal transplant.

Part of your evaluation is a percutaneous renal biopsy. The procedure goes without difficulty, and an adequate specimen is obtained. Glomerulonephritis, chronic, is the microscopic diagnosis. Few intact glomeruli are seen. One comment concerns you. A section of arterial wall is seen in the biopsy specimen.

When V. S. comes to your office one week after the biopsy, he looks very tired. You discuss the results of your various tests and list the reasonable long-term options available for V. S. to consider. Then you re-examine him. As you feared, there is a new bruit over the right kidney, which convinces you that V. S. has a post-biopsy A-V fistula. These are common occurrences after percutaneous biopsy of either the liver or kidneys, but they generally close spontaneously and rarely cause enough turbulent flow to produce bruits. With the report of arterial wall in the biopsy specimen, you worry that the fistula V. S. has will not close. You add this information to the rest you have told V. S., and he decides to think things over.

He returns a week later short of breath and looking ghastly. His bruit is still present and may even be louder. He wants the fistula occluded but is not yet able to face dialysis or renal transplantation. You admit him for right renal angiography and possible occlusion of the fistula using angiographic techniques. Three films from a selective right renal angiogram are shown on the following page. They were taken at 1.5, 2.5 and 6 seconds after the start of the contrast medium injection. What do you see?

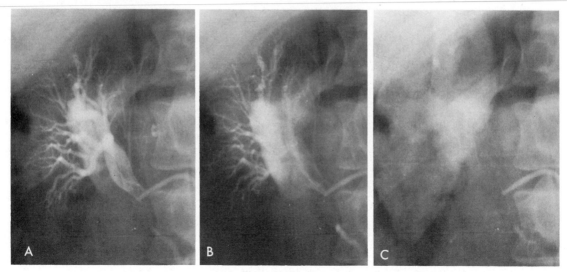

Figure 5–2a, b, c

There is dense filling of the right renal vein on the mid-arterial phase film, which is even more pronounced one second later. The inferior vena cava is faintly seen on the final film. The intrarenal arteries show changes typical of an end-stage kidney. They taper abruptly and are somewhat tortuous, and there is marked pruning of the peripheral branches. The actual fistula site cannot be seen on this run or on others in additional positions, and it was decided not to attempt percutaneous occlusion under such circumstances.

V. S. is disappointed but does come to grips with his renal problems, asking to be entered in the transplant program. He finally has some luck because a compatible donor shows up in a matter of days. No one ahead of him on the list can use this donor, so about eight weeks after you first saw him V. S. has a new kidney. Nearly a record time. When his own kidneys were removed, the A-V fistula was still wide open and it looked as if it would never close spontaneously.

P. R. is a wealthy 17 year old ne'er-do-well whose judgment and perspective are distorted by an unlimited allowance and an absence of parental guidance. Actually, as his pediatrician since birth, you are probably one of the few people he trusts and confides in. In the past several years you have seen him through numerous scrapes, both physical and legal. He is in his greatest fix now. A few weeks ago he was shot in the back by a farmer who found him harvesting cherries by moonlight. The buckshot felled P. R., and the police and an ambulance arrived simultaneously. When you reached the holding cell of the country hospital, P. R. was not exhibiting his usual degree of bravado. He had innumerable soft tissue wounds on his back, most of which were superficial, but several on the right flank that had penetrated much more deeply. P. R. had hematuria, and an excretory urogram showed several pellets to be in his right kidney, which was enlarged and had diminished function. You admitted P. R. to the prison ward of the hospital. Over a few days the hematuria subsided and P. R. seemed on the mend. His legal problems persisted, however, since the farmer was determined to prosecute P. R. for stealing cherries. Once he was ready to leave the hospital, his family lawyer posted bail and P. R., only slightly chastened, went free.

It is five weeks later when you see him again. He has developed gross hematuria, feels weak and is really scared. An excretory urogram shows no function on the right. You call a urologist, who hears the story, examines P. R. and reviews the two urograms. He thinks a nephrectomy is almost certainly necessary but requests a renal angiogram to get a better idea of what he will face at surgery, since he is concerned that the recent gunshot injury will make dissection difficult. Three films from the angiogram are shown. The first is from an aortic injection and the second two are from a selective right renal angiogram. Both you and the urologist are surprised when the radiologist reviews the films with you. What do you see?

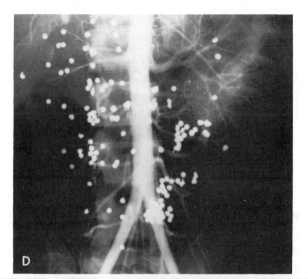

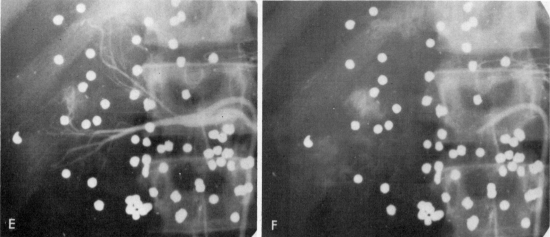

Figure 5-2d, e, f

The innumerable metallic pellets are easily seen. The aorta and left renal artery and intrarenal circulation are normal. The striking abnormality is the abrupt tapering of the right renal artery and the paucity of intrarenal branches. The selective angiogram demonstrates that the intrarenal arterial branching is markedly reduced, and there are amorphous collections of contrast material. You postulate that the kidney suffered diffuse massive trauma and is now bleeding from the disrupted parenchyma.

P. R. has a nephrectomy two days later. The operation is difficult because of obliteration of normal tissue planes but is accomplished without untoward occurrence. The kidney is completely shattered and necrotic. Histologically, the renal capsule and some blood vessels are the only recognizable parts of the kidney.

P. R. develops an aspiration pneumonia after surgery and has a rather stormy postoperative course. But, rather soon, P. R. is better, his legal problems solved, and he is whisked off by his guilt-ridden father to Bora Bora to recuperate in the sun. You wonder what will happen next.

Another approach to therapy in this situation is transcatheter embolic occlusion of the right renal artery. A variety of materials are available for this purpose, and it is a relatively simple procedure that can be done at the time of the initial angiogram. The object of such a procedure would be to non-operatively control the hemorrhage by occlusion of the renal blood supply. This approach would not save the kidney but can avoid the need for rather difficult surgery.

The unfortunate C. W. was accosted by two thugs on his way home from a late party. Unwisely, he resisted and was shot in the right flank. When he is brought to the emergency room, he is somewhat agitated and in pain, but his vital signs are stable. There is an entrance wound in the right lumbar triangle and no exit wound. While the location of the wound alone would be enough to make you suspect renal trauma, his urine is obviously bloody and you order an intravenous urogram. The preliminary film is illustrated.

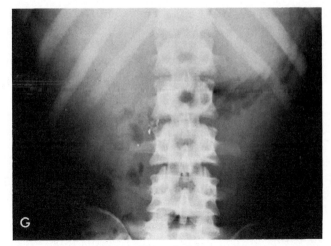

Figure 5–2g

Neither renal outline is well seen, and the right psoas margin is not at all seen. These findings may be fortuitous, but there is no mistaking the metallic fragments adjacent to the spine. The next film is obtained 10 minutes after the contrast medium injection. What do you see?

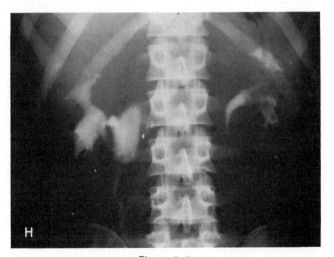

Figure 5–2h

Again, the renal outlines are not well seen, but this film was taken after the time of the maximal nephrogram. The left collecting structures are normal. On the right, the renal pelvis is distorted and there is a large, irregular contrast medium collection medial to the kidney. The bullet has apparently transversed the renal pelvis, and there is extravasation of contrast material and urine from the bullet hole.

Because of injury to the renal pelvis and a faintly positive peritoneal tap, early exploratory surgery with both a urologist and general surgeon in attendance is decided upon. At surgery, there is no significant intraperitoneal injury, but there is sizeable retroperitoneal hematoma. The kidney itself is undamaged, but the renal pelvis has a laceration, which is surgically repaired, and the perinephric space is drained.

Renal pelvic lacerations may occur with any penetrating trauma and may be seen in combination with trauma to the renal parenchyma. The treatment is generally surgical repair and drainage. The longer the duration of extravasation, the more difficult the repair becomes, so early surgery is advisable.

W. B. is waiting for a bus when suddenly he hears a burglar alarm and then gunshots. A nearby jewelry store is being robbed, and the police have arrived. Realizing he is in the cross fire, he ducks behind a mailbox only to be hit by a ricocheting bullet.

When brought to the emergency room his vital signs are stable. He complains of flank pain on the left. The entrance wound is in the costovertebral angle on the left and there is no exit wound. While his urine is clear, the nature of the injury makes you decide to order an intravenous urogram. Here is the 10 minute film. What do you think?

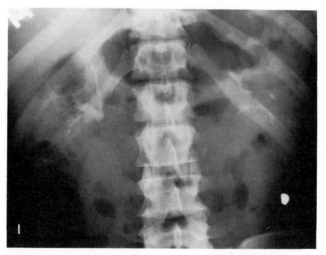

Figure 5–2i

Both kidneys excrete contrast material. The bullet lies just above the iliac crest. The left transverse process of L-2 has been fractured, giving you an idea of the course of the bullet. The left psoas margin is obliterated, and the lower pole of the left kidney is indistinct. The axis of the left kidney is more vertical than one would expect. There is no extravasation of contrast material. The findings are those of a perirenal retroperitoneal bleeding.

W. B.'s prior films become available in a few hours, and there is an old intravenous urogram, which helps to confirm that these observations are significant.

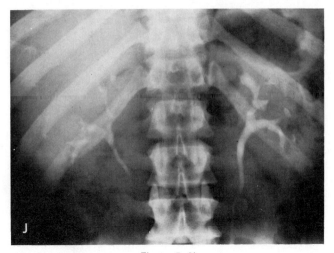

Figure 5–2j

The absence of hematuria does not totally exclude a renal parenchymal injury, but W. B. declines exploratory surgery or angiography and any further diagnostic procedures, such as a CT scan or ultrasound, which would confirm your impression of perirenal bleeding. He is admitted for observation and is discharged after an uneventful three day stay. He is rather proud of his wound and asks for a copy of his x-ray to take home.

N. M.

N. M. has a penchant for picking violent companions, and her current suitor is no exception. He stabs her in the back when he catches her kissing another man without bothering to find out that the object of her affection is her own brother. The wound doesn't hurt very much, and N. M. comes to the emergency room only when she sees blood in her urine. Indeed, the wound is not impressive. It is just below the 12th rib on the left about four inches off midline. A probe, however, goes in at least four inches and N. M. says the knife her boyfriend used has an eight inch long blade that is only half an inch wide. You are not sure what part of the urinary tract has been entered, and so you order an intravenous urogram. The preliminary film and one taken at 10 minutes are shown. What are your observations?

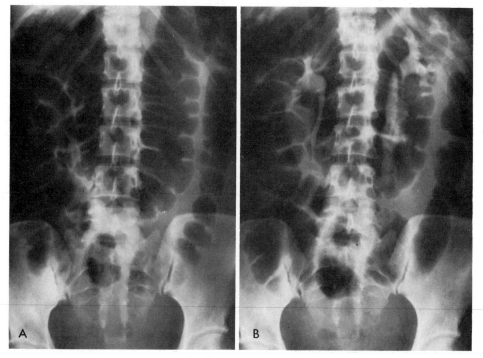

Figure 5–3a, b

The preliminary film demonstrates marked colon gas and a lesser amount of small bowel gas. This could be a simple ileus pattern, but you wonder just how far the blade did penetrate. N. M. is quite slim, and it could have easily entered the peritoneal cavity from the back. No other abnormalities are seen. On the 10 minute film, however, there are more specific findings. The right kidney and ureter are normal. The left kidney is functioning, but contrast material is extravasating from the proximal ureter and tracking in the retroperitoneal tissue planes. The kidney itself is normal. It is not possible to determine from this examination whether the ureter is lacerated or completely transected, though no contrast is seen in the distal ureter.

There is no clinical evidence of injury to other organs, and the urologist and surgeon decide to explore the stab wound along its course and do whatever repair is needed to the ureter. A rather small ureteric laceration is found which was apparently at the point of deepest penetration of the knife blade. N. M. does well with stenting of the ureter and drainage and goes home 10 days later.

When she returns for a follow-up visit four weeks later, you are shocked to learn she has married her violent boyfriend. No doubt you'll be seeing her again.

Injury to the ureter can be investigated by intravenous urography, as in this case. The laceration to the ureter is demonstrated by prograde extravasation of contrast medium. Retrograde pyelograde is an alternate approach that carries greater morbidity and complexity in this setting, but may be needed if the point of injury is not defined by the intravenous urogram. Another approach would be an antegrade pyelogram with percutaneous stenting and urinary diversion.

CASE 5–4:

D. H., MISS J. B. AND MR. R. D.

D. H. has always been deathly afraid of the broncos that his father trains for rodeo use, but at age 27 he has mastered the mechanical bucking horse in a western bar. One night, full of beer and bravado, he takes up a dare from his younger brother to mount a real bronco. They go to one of his father's small training rings where D. H. mounts a partially tamed stallion. He is thrown almost immediately and lands astride the railing and then falls into the ring. Too scared to move, he is trampled by the frightened horse until his brother, also rather incapacitated by beer, is able to distract and calm the animal.

D. H. has innumerable bumps and bruises as well as a few lacerations that need stitching. His major complaint, however, is pelvic pain, especially on urination. When his urine is bloody, you wonder if his straddle type injury caused a urethral disruption. After bone films of the pelvis reveal no fractures and a limited urogram demonstrates normal kidneys, you do a retrograde urethrogram. This is also normal, so a catheter is placed in the bladder and a cystogram is performed under fluoroscopic control. What do you see on this film?

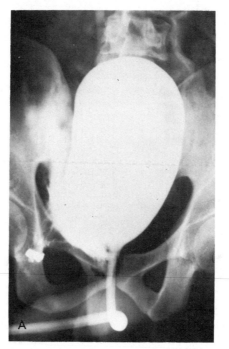

Figure 5–4a

The bladder is quite distended. On the right, there is extravasation of contrast material which is shaggy and ill-defined and does not outline bowel loops. This is contrast material tracking in retroperitoneal tissue planes and is the typical appearance of extraperitoneal bladder rupture.

D. H. recovers rather rapidly and has no complications. He knows he has been fortunate and seems quite sheepish about his foolish behavior. Perhaps he has learned from his experience.

The classic straddle injury usually involves the bulbous urethra, often crushing it. In this case, D. H. was spared such an injury but sustained a bladder rupture confined to the extraperitoneal space about the bladder, a much simpler problem. Urethrography is clearly of importance in the separation of these two entities and should be performed before catheterization if there is clinical concern about bladder injury. The cystogram can then often demonstrate location of a bladder laceration, though it should be remembered that a laceration can be present in the face of a normal cystogram. Apparently some lacerations seal over enough to prevent leakage of contrast material into the retroperitoneal or peritoneal spaces.

Miss J. B. and her boyfriend planned to spend the weekend in White Sands, New Mexico, at the dune buggy races but on the way there, he headed cross country to shorten the trip. Soon after leaving the highway they went through a gully too fast and rolled the buggy. The rollbar went over J. B.'s lower abdomen, causing immediate, severe pain. It took an hour or so for her boyfriend to bring help, and when Miss J. B. arrives at the emergency room she has a very tender abdomen and says she passed some bloody urine. The mark where the rollbar hit is easily seen on the lower abdomen, and from its location it seems much more likely that J. B. has a bladder injury than a renal one. When a catheter is placed, very bloody urine returns, further strengthening your suspicion. You order a cystogram and watch while the radiologist gently injects dilute contrast material under fluoroscopic control. You don't need the overhead film to tell you what has happened. What type of injury has occurred in Miss J. B.?

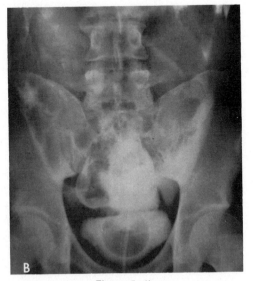

Figure 5–4b

A large Foley catheter is inflated in the bladder. The bladder is opacified and has no obvious intrinsic abnormality. However, above the bladder, contrast medium outlines loops of bowel and, in fact, is seen around bowel loops throughout the abdomen. Collections of contrast medium are seen in the recesses and gutters of the peritoneal cavity, including "dog ears" just above and lateral to the bladder. All these observations confirm your impression of an intraperitoneal rupture of the bladder. Before surgery, you request an intravenous urogram to make sure the kidneys are not injured. What do you see on this 10 minute film?

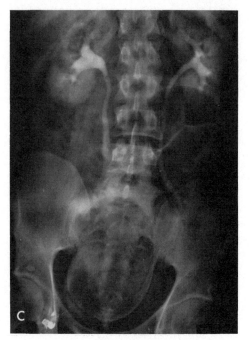

Figure 5–4c

The kidneys and upper collecting systems are normal. The ureters can be followed to the pelvic brim. Contrast medium is again seen extravasating from the dome of the bladder.

At surgery, you find a 4 cm laceration in the dome of the bladder. Repair goes well and J. B. is soon riding around in her new dune buggy.

Mr. R. D. is brought into your office by his brother who has just extracted him from the local drunk tank. Mr. R. D. has nothing to say, but his brother tells you that R. D., who is 59, has been missing for 12 days, is an alcoholic and has apparently been on a binge for most of that time. The brother is worried because R. D. seems bloated and has mentioned some pain in his abdomen.

When you examine Mr. R. D., there are a few bruises on his abdomen. He is quite distended, has no bowel sounds and is tender to palpation. The tenderness is diffuse but seems more marked in the lower abdomen. Sure Mr. R. D. has something wrong with him, but at a loss about its nature, you order an abdominal series, urinalysis and routine blood work. The supine film from the abdominal series is illustrated. What does it tell you?

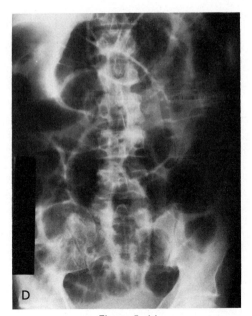

Figure 5-4d

There is rather marked distension of both the small and large bowel. The distension is symmetrical throughout, so a profound ileus is the most likely diagnosis. Decubitus and upright films are also consistent with this idea. If you are observant, you have wondered about the loss of fat planes in the pelvis and the separation of bowel loops in the lower abdomen, which suggests fluid.

In effect, the films have not helped you greatly in a decision of what to do next, though they have added to your certainty that something is really wrong with Mr. R. D. The laboratory reports its findings. There is microscopic hematuria and a moderate leukocytosis. Not very helpful, but you question R. D. more carefully about his bruises and other experiences since his disappearance. He is quite unsure about his odyssey but thinks he was roughed up and robbed one evening. Some young toughs jumped on his abdomen while he was sleeping in an alley. In conjunction with the hematuria, this makes you wonder about a bladder injury, so you plan to do a cystogram, intravenous urogram and barium studies, in that order, as needed.

The urine that drains out when the catheter is placed for the cystogram is pink-tinged. About 150 cc of contrast material is instilled into the bladder under fluoroscopic control. What do you see on the film on the following page, taken after filling?

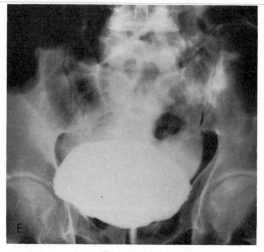

Figure 5–4e

The bladder is moderately distended and rather smooth-walled, and no filling defects are seen. Above the bladder is a less well-defined collection of contrast material. Where do you think this lies? Though its lateral margins are sharply defined, the superior aspect of the collection fades off. On the left, you should wonder if it surrounds a loop of bowel. The contrast medium is then drained from the bladder, and another film taken. Where do you think the contrast medium that remains is located?

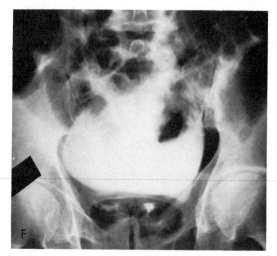

Figure 5–4f

A very small amount of contrast material remains in the collapsed bladder. The remainder is in the recesses of the peritoneal cavity, indicating that the bladder had indeed been ruptured through the peritoneum.

Mr. R. D. was taken to surgery after lengthy discussion about what should be done, since his injury was of indeterminate age. A bladder laceration about 6 cm long was found and repaired. All cultures of his abdominal fluid were sterile, so Mr. R. D. gets off rather easily this time.

M. S., J. M. AND J. C.

No one is ever sure how M. S., an experienced farm hand, managed to get himself entangled with a huge combine during the wheat harvest, but he does and is brought into the emergency room with an array of bumps, bruises and fractures. As you sort out his various complaints, the most serious ones relate to his pelvis. He has marked swelling and tenderness over his pubic symphysis and has gross hematuria. You order appropriate films. The AP of the pelvis is demonstrated. What do you see and what are your concerns?

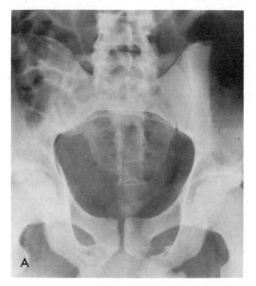

Figure 5–5a

There are comminuted fractures of both inferior pubic rami with marked displacement of some of the fracture fragments. There is slight diastasis of the pubic symphysis and a fracture involving the right acetabulum. There is probably an acetabular fracture on the left. The fat planes on the right are obscured, and there is a soft tissue mass along the right pelvic wall. The sacroiliac joints are asymmetrical, with separation on the right.

Such severe pelvic trauma should make you worry about injury to the bladder or urethra. In this case, the worry is made greater by your knowledge that the patient has gross hematuria. After consultation with a urologist you decide to do a retrograde urethrogram and cystogram. A film from the urethrogram is shown. What do you see?

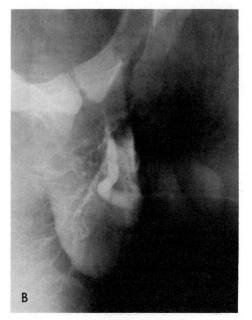

Figure 5–5b

A small catheter has been introduced into the urethral meatus, and contrast material has been gently injected under fluoroscopic control. The pendulous urethra is normal, but there is laceration of the membranous urethra with extravasation of contrast material into the soft tissues of the perineum. Though M. S. can urinate, you cannot pass a catheter into the bladder, so that cystogram is done as a late film after an intravenous urogram. What do you see on this AP film?

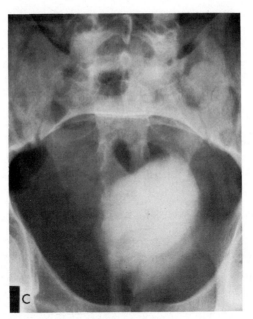

Figure 5–5c

The bladder is elevated from the pelvic floor and is displaced to the left and up, most likely by hemorrhage from the numerous pelvic fractures M. S. has suffered.

M. S. has a prolonged hospital course because of his many fractures, but the urethral injury heals well and M. S. has no stricture when he finally leaves the rehabilitation center in time for the next wheat harvest.

You have just discharged M. S. when J. M. and J. C. arrive almost simultaneously in the emergency room.

J. M. is an old car buff without much in the way of mechanical commonsense. He loves to tinker with his cars and continually gets into one sort of scrape or another. This time, his wife calls to say she is bringing him in because a jack slipped, causing the rear end of a lovely, large Pierce Arrow to fall on his pelvis. With the help of the next door neighbor, she has extricated J. M. He is faint and in pain, but has refused the ambulance she thinks he needs.

When they arrive, J. M. is obviously in shock and cannot urinate. You order films of the pelvis. What do you see on the film that is shown?

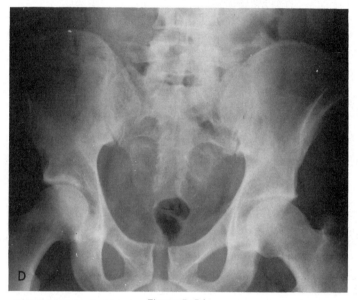

Figure 5–5d

The most dramatic abnormality is separation of the symphysis pubis. One fracture or separation in the ring structure usually means that there is another, and you can see that there is a fracture through the left sacrum. The soft tissues within the pelvis, especially near the symphysis pubis, should draw your attention at this point, since soft tissue injury often accompanies such pelvic fractures. There is asymmetry of the perivesical fat planes, and the bladder seems to be elevated. This is a non-specific finding, since while bleeding can do this, so can urine extravasating from either the bladder or the urethra. You decide to order an intravenous urogram next. If J. M. still can't void when that examination is complete, you plan to go ahead with a retrograde urethrogram.

A single film from the urogram is shown. What do you think?

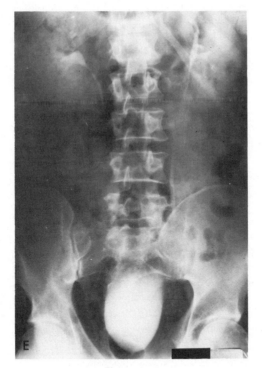

Figure 5–5e

Both kidneys function and the upper collecting systems are normal. The ureters, where seen, are also normal. The bladder is elevated and has an elongated shape, which is a deformity typical of a perivisceral hematoma. No extravasation of contrast material is seen, but this does not completely exclude a bladder laceration. J. M. still cannot void, and you go ahead with the retrograde urethrogram. When the Foley catheter is passed gently into the distal urethra, you get back a bloody drainage. Water soluble contrast material is carefully and gently injected under fluoroscopic control, and the radiologist takes several films. One is illustrated on the following page. What is your diagnosis?

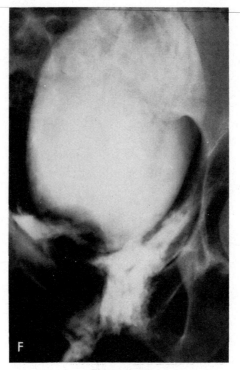

Figure 5–5f

Contrast medium has extravasated into the pelvic soft tissues along the posterior urethra and at the bladder base. In view of the pelvic injury, a rupture of the posterior urethra is the first diagnosis you should entertain. Fractures involving the pubic symphysis also disrupt the puboprostatic ligament, allowing a shearing force to develop at the junction of the membranous and prostatic urethras when the prostate moves. Such a force can easily lead to a posterior urethral rupture. Since the rupture occurs above the urogenital diaphragm, blood is not seen in the perineal tissues. All the bleeding and extravasated urine is contained between the urogenital diaphragm and the pelvic fascial planes.

You call in a urologist, since complications including strictures, fistulae and impotence are frequent with such ruptures. J. M. signs out of the hospital eight days later to attend a Rolls Royce auction in England. You wonder what will happen but hear nothing for months. Finally, you get a postcard from Brighton saying that they are staying permanently in England. Too many lovely old cars, it seems.

Mr. J. C., on the other hand, is a sad story. He lives in halfway homes for the mentally ill and generally manages to get by on odd jobs. Periodically, he becomes overwhelmed by life, and if someone doesn't notice his increased nervousness, he invariably does something to himself that requires hospitalization. He has been admitted for drug overdoses, for a swallowed razor blade and for a burn that needed skin grafting. This time he is having hematuria when he comes to the office. You comfort him and calm him down, promising he will be cared for and kept safe. He finally confesses that he passed a Phillips screwdriver up his urethra several times until he caused the bleeding. You are not particularly surprised, but you need to know how serious the injury is. Once again, you request a urethrogram. Two films are illustrated. What do you think?

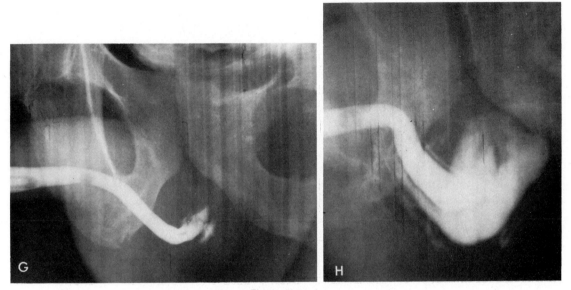

Figure 5-5g, h

The initial film shows the tip of the catheter in the distal bulbous urethra. There is an ovoid air bubble near it. The contrast medium column stops abruptly in the proximal bulbous urethra, and contrast material is seen extravasating into the tissues. The second film shows further extravasation into the soft tissues. Some penile veins are also opacified. Once again, you call in a urologist to assist you. Mr. J. C. responds well to conservative treatment for his anterior urethral laceration, but his psychiatric problems have become severe and it is months before he is able to return to a halfway house.

Urethral injuries are uncommon in the female except those caused during childbirth. However, severe pelvic fractures can disrupt the female urethra, and this should be considered in such trauma. The male anterior urethra can receive both blunt and penetrating injuries. Since strictures are as important to avoid as fistulae, prompt diagnosis and appropriate therapy assume great importance. Retrograde urethrography is indicated in most situations, though occasionally a prograde voiding study after intravenous urogram will provide enough information. When urethral trauma is a possibility, a urethrogram should be performed before attempts are made to catheterize the bladder. Such manipulation can aggravate a urethral injury.

MRS. M. L. AND MR. J. S. E.

Mrs. M. L. is an obese, shaky, 78 year old woman who is stubborn enough to refuse assistance in her daily tasks. She is returning from the farmers market with her arms full of groceries when she loses her balance, lurches off the sidewalk and is grazed by a city bus. She falls heavily on her left side, scattering her groceries. The bus driver calls for a city ambulance, and Mrs. M. L. is finally persuaded to go to the emergency room.

When you examine her, she mentions some pain deep in her back on the left. Her description is not very helpful, but deep palpation does increase her distress and there seems to be some fullness in the left mid abdomen. You draw blood for laboratory studies and request abdominal films. At this point, Mrs. M. L. refuses further treatment and demands that a taxi be called for her. No amount of reasoning deters her and she departs.

You are not at all surprised to see Mrs. M. L. return the following morning. She is now in severe pain and becomes lightheaded when she stands. She is apologetic about her behavior yesterday. You again draw blood and send her for abdominal radiographs. The supine film is demonstrated. What do you see?

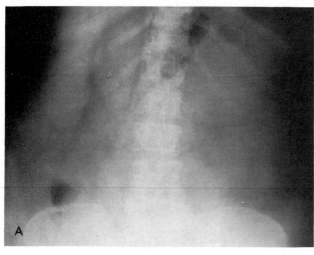

Figure 5–6a

This film is of limited diagnostic value both because the patient is obese and for technical reasons. Several observations should be made, however. The abdomen is nearly gasless, but the stomach, which does contain some gas, is displaced to the right. The left psoas margin is not seen but then neither is the right. The entire left abdomen has a very homogeneous, gray look, and you are concerned about splenic injury. The remainder of the abdominal films do not add any more useful information. The laboratory reports that the hematocrit is 28 mg%, and you are even more concerned about bleeding, since yesterday's level was 39 mg%.

You tell Mrs. M. L. that you think that she is bleeding somewhere in her abdomen, possibly from a damaged spleen. CT seems the most efficient way to look for bleeding in Mrs. M. L., so you arrange for an emergency scan. The study is performed first without any contrast material, and the radiologist calls to say that the spleen is normal but there is an extensive adjacent abnormality. He plans to inject some contrast material and repeat selected sections. You go over to the CT unit to see the study. Two films done prior to injection of contrast material are demonstrated. What do you see?

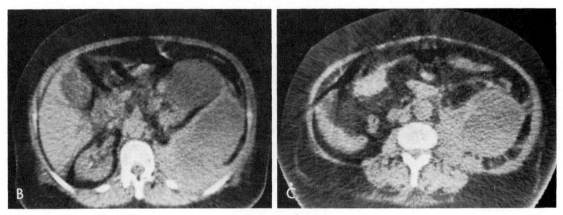

Figure 5–6b, c

The higher section includes the right lobe of the liver with the gallbladder and the right kidney. On the left, there is a large mass that is displacing the left kidney ventrally. The mass has an area of lower attenuation laterally. The left kidney is abnormal with a low attenuation, rounded mass protruding from its lateral margin. The lower section shows a round mass intimately involved with the left psoas muscle that has a lower attenuation centrally than peripherally. You are sure you have located the site of Mrs. M. L.'s bleeding, though the actual source is not apparent.

The contrast study is now completed, and the two parts of the examinations are compared. A single section from the contrast examination is illustrated on the following page. It was done at about the same level as the first non-contrast section. What are your observations?

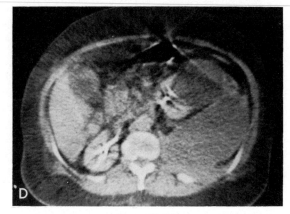

Figure 5–6d

The kidneys are now opacified, and the collecting systems are seen. The very anterior position of the left kidney is again demonstrated, and the mass on its lateral border is clearly a cyst.

Since Mrs. M. L. is not a good surgical risk and has an extensive retroperitoneal hematoma without an obvious source, a course of blood replacement and watchful waiting is decided upon. Over the next few days she improves, with gradual decrease in pain and no indication of recurrent bleeding. When she is ready to be discharged, you try to tell her to get assistance in her chores, but she reasserts her independence and goes home in a huff.

Of the diagnostic procedures available to evaluate Mrs. M. L.'s problem, CT was chosen for a variety of reasons. Splenic trauma or a retroperitoneal bleed seemed the most logical diagnostic possibilities. While ultrasound can study both areas, in Mrs. M. L., obesity and pain were likely to limit the success of examination. CT, on the other hand, is generally more satisfactory in the obese patient. This case demonstrates the ability of CT to examine the retroperitoneum and demonstrate its various compartments. The normal appearance of the spleen does not exclude a splenic injury, but an isotope spleen scan was normal and Mrs. M. L. steadfastly refused angiography, the most accurate means of excluding subtle splenic injury.

Mr. J. S. E. is a 28 year old fellow who functions in the twilight zone between a frankly criminal life and a reasonably average existence. He has come to the emergency room in the past for assorted stabbings and gunshot wounds, but this is the first time he has been seriously injured. Even his arrival is dramatic. A man races into the reception area and grabs a gurney. The receptionist tries to ask what he wants, but he simply pushes the gurney out the door, and by the time she and a guard get to the door, the gurney is being returned with a body on it. When the man pushing the gurney sees the guard, he dashes for a van, which immediately roars off into the darkness.

J. S. E. is in shock and is lying in a pool of blood. He is rapidly stripped, blood is drawn and intravenous lines are started. Examination reveals a bullet wound in the left midaxillary line at about T10. It is clear that an exploratory laparotomy is necessary in short order, but since J. S. E. responds to intravenous fluids, you get a limited number of films on the way to surgery. A chest film does not show a pneumothorax or intrathoracic hemorrhage. Abdominal film shows a bullet adjacent to L4, and when a lateral film shows the bullet to be posterior, you get a limited excretory urogram. One film is illustrated. What are your observations?

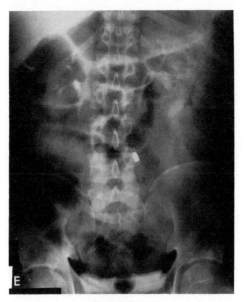

Figure 5–6e

There is a slight scoliosis of the lumbar spine with the convexity to the right. The bullet is lying against the left side at L4 in this projection with its nose pointing cephalad. The vertebral body is intact. The right kidney is functioning normally. The left is also functioning, but the concentration of contrast material is less than that on the right and the collecting system may be a bit full. Neither ureter is well seen.

Mr. J. S. E. goes to surgery. On opening his abdomen, a mixture of blood and bowel contents is found. A splenectomy is performed because the spleen is shattered. Four holes in the splenic flexure of the colon are closed. The small bowel is intact, but arteries in the root of the mesentery have been transected with extension of the hematoma into the retroperitoneum on the left. You make the needed repairs and satisfy yourself that the left ureter is not transected. The bullet is inaccessible and, after doing a diverting colostomy, you close the abdomen and place J. S. E. on antibiotics. Youth pays off and J. S. E. has an uneventful ten day rest in the hospital.

Nearly nine weeks after discharge, J. S. E. comes to your office with severe muscle spasms in his back. These are not incapacitating, but he wants something done. Physical examination reveals only some deep tenderness over his lower back. He does have an elevated white count. You request abdominal films. A detail from one is illustrated. What pertinent observations can you make?

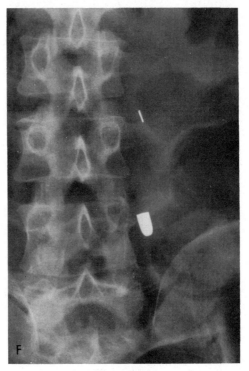

Figure 5–6f

You notice that the bullet has changed its orientation. Its nose now points caudad. You also wonder about the superior end plate of L4. It seems less well defined than on earlier films. You suspect that J. S. E. has both a psoas abscess and osteomyelitis and want to work him up more thoroughly, but he has some "business" to do, so he leaves, promising to return when he has more time.

You see him nine days later, by which time he can hardly stand straight. He is more than willing to be hospitalized, since he has taken care of his "business" and wants to be out of sight. On admission you order lumbar spine films. What do you see on the x-ray shown?

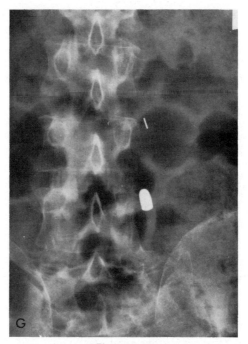

Figure 5-6g

The bullet has once again changed its orientation, and now you are sure that there is destruction on L4 adjacent to the bullet. To confirm this, a CT scan is obtained. What does this section through L4 show?

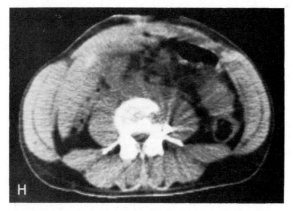

Figure 5-6h

The bullet is the very high attenuation object giving off a "spray" artifact that obscures detail in the left psoas muscle. More dramatic is the large defect in the vertebral body itself. The left psoas is larger than the right. Putting the whole story together, you are sure J. S. E. has a psoas abscess. The space filled with pus around the bullet allows it to tumble. There is also osteomyelitis of L4. The psoas abscess is drained, and appropriate antibiotics are started. Mr. J. S. E. becomes rather impatient with the time he is spending in the hospital, but doesn't sign out as you fear. Apparently his "business" has not yet settled down.

Months after discharge you read that he drowned while trying to transfer drugs from a coastal steamer to a smaller boat. Somehow, such an end seemed inevitable.

Late infections following penetrating trauma are surprisingly uncommon considering the presence of necrotic tissue and the possibilities for contamination. In this case the "tumbing" of the bullet showed that it was in a cavity, and CT was particularly useful in defining the extent of the problem, showing both the bony and soft tissue components of the infection.

CHAPTER

6

EXTREMITIES

INTRODUCTION

Extremity trauma is very common in any emergency room. Fractures and dislocations are among the most frequent injuries. Soft tissue trauma usually accompanies skeletal trauma but often can be adequately evaluated without the use of radiographs. On the other hand, serious vascular injury can accompany fractures. Good examples of this are popliteal artery lacerations and occlusions associated with shearing injury to the knee and the anterior compartment syndromes that may accompany severe fractures of the tibia and fibula. Ligamentous and cartilaginous tears also occur with fractures. These may need arthrography or other radiographic studies.

Both high and low velocity penetrating injuries occur in the extremities. Again, vascular injury is a serious concern, and angiography may be indicated. In other situations, the foreign body that produced the penetrating injury must be identified and localized for removal. Delayed complications of penetrating wounds, such as infection or vascular sequelae, may also need radiographic evaluation.

Since soft tissue injury to the extremities is exceedingly varied, the radiologist and attending physician should use an innovative, imaginative approach to these problems. Routine radiographs of an arm or a leg may suffice but often will not answer the clinical question of greatest concern. Radiographic consultation can hasten the choice of the correct diagnostic study.

MISS R. S.

A roller skaters' convention is under way in Central Park, and you have already seen scrapes and bruises, fractures and a possible concussion among the conventioneers when Miss R. S. shows up with a dramatic, if rather minor, roller skating injury. She had been warming up for a dance competition by skating around the reservoir when she fell. Unfortunately, she was holding her house keys in her right hand, and one penetrated her palm on the ventral surface and is bulging the skin on the dorsal surface of her hand. The key cannot be withdrawn easily. The injury is not very painful except when the key is moved. Before you attempt to remove it, you get radiographs to see the exact position of the key and look for bony injury.

The AP and lateral films are demonstrated. What are your observations?

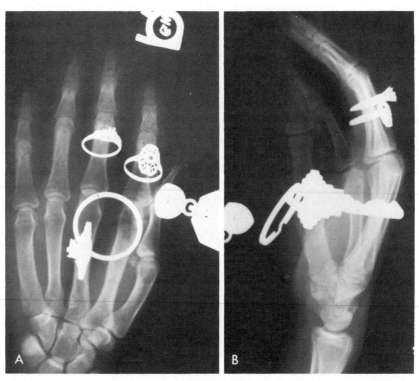

Figure 6–1a, b

The key penetrates the hand between the third and fourth metacarpals. No bony injury is demonstrated, though the key does obscure part of the third metacarpal.

The key comes out easily once the area is anesthetized. No major bleeding occurs, and inspection of the wound and hand confirms that no ligamentous injury has occurred. After cleaning and dressing the wound, you send Miss R. S. off with a suggestion to be more careful when she goes skating. She might not be so lucky another time.

J. T.

Foreign bodies come in all shapes and sizes and carry highly varied degrees of significance. You thought you had seen everything from pediatric ingestions to the perverse, but J. T. provides a new, if obvious, problem. He is a professional painter who routinely uses high pressure paint sprayers but, when the rigging on his scaffold slips, he injects paint into the soft tissues of his thumb. The entrance wound is ragged but quite small, and the tip of the thumb is swollen, red and very tender. You doubt there has been bony injury but order an x-ray to make sure. What do you see on the lateral film illustrated?

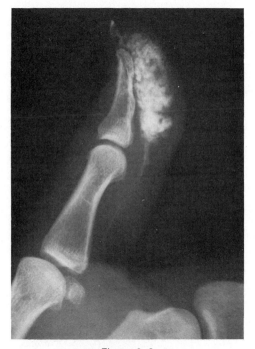

Figure 6–2

The bones are normal in this projection. The paint has spread diffusely through the soft tissues of the distal thumb and either is dissecting along a muscle plane or has entered a vein. The paint is radiopaque in this case. When you ask J. T. what sort of paint he is using, it proves to be white lead exterior house paint in an oil base. Non-leaded paints would not produce such a dramatic radiograph.

Since you are concerned about the viability of the skin over the paint, you refer J. T. to a plastic surgeon specializing in hand problems. Conservative therapy is used, and later you hear that a small skin graft was needed but otherwise J. T. did well.

MS. B. R.

Ms. B. R. is a 23 year old apprentice glazier who is brought to the emergency room by ambulance. Her right ankle is wrapped in a large dressing, and one of the ambulance attendants is compressing her right femoral artery to decrease bleeding. You unwrap her leg and find a very nasty gash that goes down to the bone just above the ankle. The Achilles tendon is undoubtedly severed. Apparently, a very large sheet of plate glass shattered, and a jagged fragment struck her leg. You wonder about bits of glass in the wound and order x-rays both to look for glass and to make sure there is no fracture. Is there any glass in the wound?

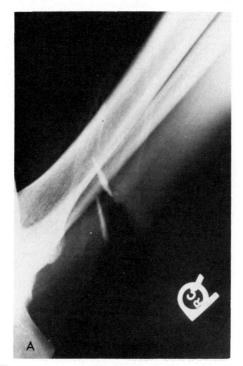

Figure 6–3a

There are two sizable pieces of glass and at least one small fragment seen in this projection. An additional view demonstrated several more small fragments. The bones are not fractured, but the Achilles tendon is severed and retracted. Clinically, the circulation to the foot is intact. Before repair of the laceration can be started, the glass shards must be removed, so you spend some time picking out pieces. When you can neither feel nor see any more glass, the x-rays are repeated along with a film of the recovered fragments. What do you see?

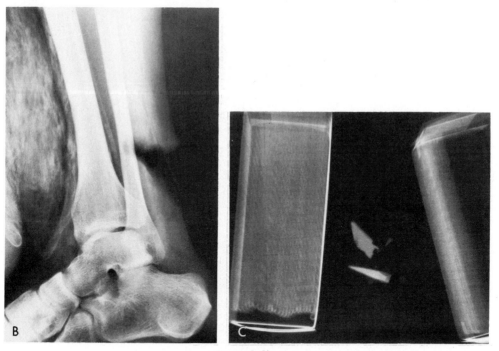

Figure 6–3b, c

The lateral film of the ankle shows no residual glass fragments. The laceration is unchanged, and the foot is now propped on a pad. The second x-ray shows the several glass fragments that you removed.

The surgical repair goes well, and Ms. B. R. goes home in five days. She is followed by her surgeon, and it is months later when she comes into the emergency room because she turned her right ankle badly playing volley ball. It is swollen but no fractures are seen on x-ray.

What do you see on the lateral film of her right ankle taken about 10 months after her initial injury?

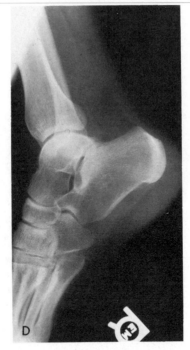

Figure 6–3d

The laceration has completely healed. The Achilles tendon has a bulbous distal end, and there is thickening of the soft tissues because of scarring. An old Achilles tendon rupture often has this appearance.

Glass is only radiopaque when it has a sufficient lead content. Glass from soft drink bottles, for example, can rarely be seen on standard radiographs. Such glass can usually be detected on xeroradiographs. Other foreign bodies, such as wood splinters, may also require xeroradiography for demonstration.

Mr. L. B. is one of your more trying patients. He is always "into" something. Recent fads have included hang gliding (he broke a leg), motor boat racing, a water and vitamin diet (he lost weight but had to be hospitalized for acute water intoxication), and "bronco busting." You feel a man of 50 should have more sense. When his wife calls to ask for an emergency appointment, she says he has been behaving oddly for the past few weeks. Some of her insulin syringes have disappeared, and she wonders if he has taken up drugs. In any case, he has a very swollen sore right arm, and she will bring him in.

When they arrive, you also find Mr. L. B.'s behavior strange. More immediately, his right arm is grotesquely swollen, red and very tender, and there are areas of crepitus. Mr. L. B. vehemently denies any kind of penetrating injury. Rather than press the issue, you order x-rays of his arm. What do you see?

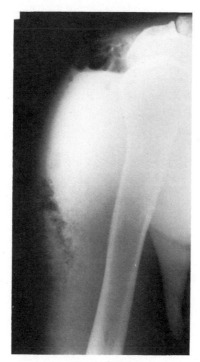

Figure 6–4

The deltoid muscle is markedly swollen, and there are many mottled lucencies throughout the area of swelling. The most obvious ones are near the shoulder, where they have coalesced, and there are several air fluid levels. The bones look normal on this and other films.

Armed with such a graphic film of a deltoid abscess, you ask Mr. L. B. again about injuries, especially penetrating ones caused by objects like needles or ice picks. A bit guiltily, he admits to "trying drugs" and being terrible with needles. It seems he kept dropping his syringe because of fear of the needle and frequently made intramuscular injections out of desperation.

Mr. L. B. is admitted to the hospital for incison and drainage of his deltoid abscess. Mercifully, he is not addicted and you later hear he is "into" skydiving.

Penetrating wounds, whether caused by needles or nails or ice picks, all carry a risk of setting up an infection deep in the soft tissues. These infections are often anaerobic. Osteomyelitis may also develop from such penetrating soft tissue injuries. Radiology generally has little role in these problems, though the nature or extent of a mass or the presence of osteomyelitis can be evaluated by radiography. If osteomyelitis is a primary concern and the soft tissues are normal, isotopic evaluation will demonstrate bony abnormality earlier than radiographs.

R. E. F. AND A. H.

R. E. F. arrives at the college infirmary looking drawn and haggard, so much so that the duty nurse puts him ahead of other waiting patients. You are somewhat surprised when you see him and find his problem is an asymptomatic, very hard lump in his mid thigh and that he feels fine. The mass is undeniably there, and it is only when you remember that a fellow member of the ice hockey team recently lost a leg to an osteogenic sarcoma that you understand why R. E. F. is so afraid. You order x-rays to get a better look at the mass. Can you reassure R. E. P. after looking at this film, which is coned down to the mid femoral shaft?

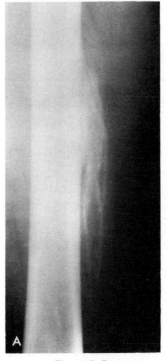

Figure 6–5a

There is a streaky calcification in the soft tissues beside the femur. What you are seeing is ossification, and the striated appearance is typical of myositis ossificans. You ask R. E. F. about recent injuries, feeling rather foolish, since he is a leading light of the ice hockey team. He reminds you that about three months ago he bruised his thigh badly in a motorcycle accident. You had taken films then and so you review them. What do you see?

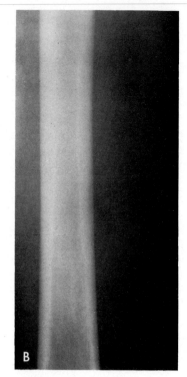

Figure 6–5b

Nothing abnormal. Myositis ossificans usually follows muscle trauma, and the ossification may be seen within weeks of the injury. It is generally somewhat streaky or striated and is usually of no clinical significance. Occasionally it may have a feathery appearance, and there may be periosteal reaction. It should be remembered that chronic neurologic problems can also lead to myositis ossificans and that there is an uncommon congenital form.

A. H. is a 69 year old man who is helping his neighbor move a bookcase. She is rather unsteady and drops her end of the bookcase without warning, causing a shelf to fall out. It strikes A. H. in the lower leg, causing severe pain and immediate reddish-blue swelling. The pain increases over the next few minutes, and A. H. is brought to your office by his neighbor. When you see him, he is unwilling to stand on his leg. You find a large, tense swelling, which you suspect is a hematoma. You order films to exclude a fracture and a prothrombin time because A. H. is on coumadin. What do you see on the AP film illustrated?

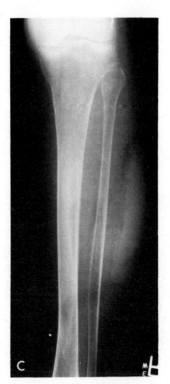

Figure 6-5c

There is no fracture, though the bones are quite demineralized. There is some vascular calcification. Most striking is the oval soft tissue mass lateral to the fibula. This is an acute hematoma.

The prothrombin is quite low at 22%. You feel this explains the remarkable hematoma that A. H. has developed from only moderate trauma. You plan to correct the overanticoagulation and otherwise treat Mr. A. H. symptomatically. You warn him about the dangers of being too chivalrous and he agrees. However, when you see him in a week he tells you his leg is much better and he is planning to help a recent widow move to his building.

There is little reason to radiograph a clinically apparent hematoma in an extremity. Hematomas are usually incidental observations seen in limbs examined to exclude a fracture. The bleeding generally obliterates tissue planes, and the hematoma is seldom as sharply defined as in this case.

CASE 6–6:

DR. G. O.

Dr. G. O., an older but still active colleague, has fallen while walking from his office to the hospital. It seems he was chatting and missed the curb as he crossed the street. Now he complains that his tight schedule is being disrupted and that he has pain around his knee and cannot extend his right leg. This leads you to suspect damage to the quadriceps tendon. You order films of the knee. What do you see?

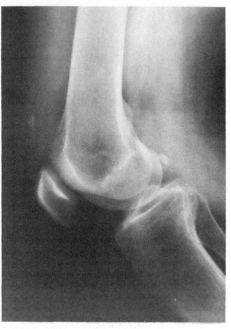

Figure 6–6

The most striking finding is the small ossified density proximal to the patella. This is ossification in the distal part of the quadriceps tendon, at the site of its insertion on the patella and is indicative of degenerative change in the tendon. The tendon has torn through the degenerated, weakened area, separating from the patella. There is also marked swelling and an effusion that is probably bloody in the suprapatellar bursa. Part of this shadow may also be blood in the tissues about the distal tendon. These findings are typical of quadriceps avulsion or rupture, though ossification or calcification of the degenerating tendon is not always seen.

Surgical repair is needed along with immobilization, but you soon see Dr. G. O. up and around, attending to his busy practice in a cast.

Tendon rupture may occur with trivial trauma if the tendon has been injured in the past or has undergone degeneration. When the trauma is minimal or not remembered, the rupture is regarded as "spontaneous." Tendon injury is usually apparent to the experienced clinician, because the involved muscle is unable to function normally. The role of radiology is limited but can exclude an associated or underlying bony abnormality.

Avid skier R. S. calls early Monday to make an appointment. Your nurse tells him to come right to the office when he says he cannot walk. As you expect, he misjudged a turn on an icy slope Saturday, fell, felt something give in his left knee and had to be carried from the hill. X-rays taken at a hospital near the slopes showed no fracture, but he still has pain on weight bearing and marked swelling. The knee feels as if it will buckle under him when he tries to walk, and Sunday evening it "froze" in a flexed position. He could only straighten it with the aid of a friend's gentle manipulation. Physical examination shows a tender, swollen knee with a large effusion, and there is a clicking sensation medially when you try to flex the knee. Though it is difficult to be sure, the tibia seems to move forward on the "drawer" maneuver. These findings suggest serious internal injury to the menisci and ligaments of the knee. You order a contrast arthrogram to better define the damage before the surgery which you suspect is indicated.

Two films from the arthrogram are shown: lateral and oblique views with stress. What is your opinion?

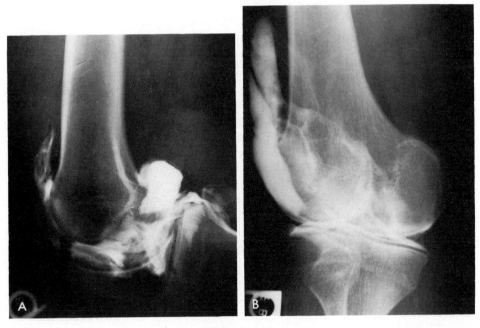

Figure 6–7a, b

The findings are quite dramatic. Remember, the contrast material introduced into the joint outlines the articular and meniscal cartilages, which appear black. The cruciate ligaments should also be seen. On the lateral view of the knee, the posterior cruciate ligament is seen as a well-defined vertical band between the femur and tibia. The anterior cruciate is not seen as a band but is rolled up in the intracondylar notch of the femur. This confirms your clinical impression of a tear of this ligament.

On the oblique view of the knee, the posterior portion of the medial meniscus and the anterior portion of the lateral meniscus are seen but not tangentially. These should be sharply defined triangular radiolucencies. Look closely at the medial meniscus. On your right, there is a thin wisp of contrast that extends into the meniscus. Now, study the spot film of this area.

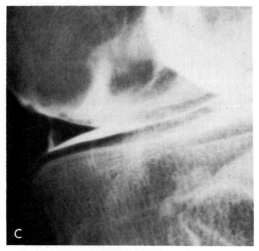

Figure 6–7c

With spot filming, the meniscus can be positioned tangentially to the x-ray beam and therefore be better examined. There is an irregular vertical band of contrast material extending from the inferior to the superior surface of the meniscus. The inner apex of the meniscus remains sharp. This is a "bucket handle" type tear. In this injury, the inner portion of the meniscus is separated from the outer portion and is free to move independently while the outer part remains normally attached at its margin. The bucket handle tear certainly explains the knee-locking episode, since the apical fragment can become fixed in a position that prevents motion in the way a door wedge holds open a door.

R. S. is dismayed that he will miss the rest of the ski season but accepts surgical correction. He is soon working out with weights, preparing for next year.

Arthrography is an excellent tool for evaluating the interior of joints. While the technique can be applied in any synovial joint, it is most often used in the larger joints, such as the knee, shoulder and hip. This technique is particularly valuable in the knee, which has a rather complex internal structure that is not visualized on plain films. The only other methods that can evaluate the cartilaginous and ligamentous structures of the knee or other joints are careful physical examination and arthroscopy, the introduction of a small endoscope into the joint which requires anesthesia and hospitalization.

J. F. is a 50 year old man whom you first saw about three weeks ago. At that time, he came to the emergency room with a wound in the left antecubital fossa and a tourniquet around his upper arm. He said he was stabbed with an ice pick when he tried to stop a barroom brawl. Though there was brisk bleeding when the tourniquet was removed, J. F. said direct pressure would stop the bleeding, and in fact 20 minutes of compression proved that to be true. Distal pulses were good and there was no hematoma. You wanted to admit J. F. for observation but he refused, so you dressed the wound and cautioned him about problems with recurrent bleeding. He left the emergency room after an interview with the police about four hours after his arrival.

There was no further trouble with the acute injury but, when J. F. began to use his arm, it was weak and his fingers were always cold. He also began to feel a continuous vibrating sensation in his arm. He comes back to your office because of these problems, and you see that the skin wound has healed well, but find his radial pulse distinctly diminished. There is also a palpable thrill over the antecubital fossa. It seems clear that J. F. has developed an arteriovenous fistula, and your opinion is confirmed by a vascular surgeon, who requests an angiogram before he attempts to repair the artery and vein.

Four films of the anteroposterior angiographic series are shown. They are taken at one, two, four and eight seconds after the start of the contrast medium injection. A lateral run was also performed. What do you see on the films shown on the following page, and why was a lateral run also made?

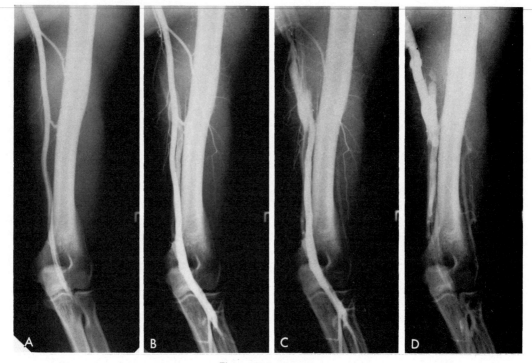

Figure 6–8a, b, c, d

At two seconds, there is already filling of a vein lying between the brachial artery and the humerus. Little arterial flow goes distally. The draining vein is distended, and there is reflux filling of veins below the elbow. The actual site of the fistula is not seen in this filming series and therefore the lateral run was performed, since precise localization of a fistula is useful to the surgeon. In J. F. the lateral run also did not demonstrate the actual fistula, probably because of the rapid, massive shunting. On both runs, however, the fistula has to be about where the entrance wound was. There is no evidence of multiple feeding arteries or draining veins, as would be seen in an arteriovenous malformation.

J. F.'s traumatic arteriovenous fistula is surgically repaired without difficulty. These lesions are not infrequent following penetrating soft tissue injuries. The communication between artery and vein causes symptoms because of high flow and because it "steals" blood from the circulation distal to it. The enlarged draining vein may feel like a pulsatile mass. In general, operative repair is indicated, though some fistulae will close spontaneously and others can be occluded by catheter embolization.

MR. A. G., MISS L. D. AND MS. W. J.

Mr. A. G. is an old gentleman who has had intermittent transient ischemic attacks for some months. At 89, he sees no reason to bother about these passing spells, but finally his granddaughter convinces him that having a real stroke would interfere with his gardening, so he agrees to an angiogram and possible carotid endarterectomy. When you explain the angiogram to him, he is intrigued by the procedure and you find him a pleasure to talk to. However, the next morning when the nurse begins to prepare him for the angiogram, he becomes cantankerous and actually tries to hit her as she shaves his groin. Upset, she drapes him hastily and, distracted, you feel a good pulse and proceed to make the arterial puncture without carefully checking your landmarks. You enter the artery on the first try, and catheter passage goes easily at first. Within a very short time, however, the artery goes into spasm, and catheter manipulation becomes difficult. You exchange the small cerebral catheter for a larger one with more torque control but still have trouble moving the catheter. Mr. A. G. senses that there is a problem and thrashes around, dislodging his drapes. You discover that the puncture site is well below the inguinal ligament, so you know you have catheterized either the deep or the superficial femoral artery. A hand injection of contrast material shows that the catheter is in the superficial femoral artery. You decide to start over on the left, and so the catheter is removed and the puncture site is compressed for 15 minutes.

All goes well from then on as far as the carotid bifurcation and arch study is concerned. Mr. A. G. calms down for most of the procedure, but after coughing he begins to complain of increasing pain in his right leg. The nurse says his peripheral pulses are good, but when she inspects the arterial puncture site, she finds an enlarging hematoma. You compress the site for another 15 minutes and the hematoma seems to stabilize, but you do a "pullout" angiogram to see what is going on. One film of the angiographic series is shown on the following page. The contrast material was injected at the aortic bifurcation. What do you see?

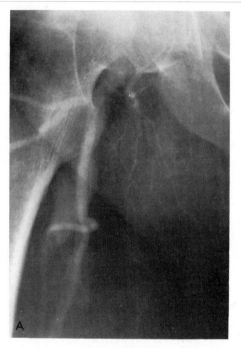

Figure 6–9a

Contrast medium is faintly seen in the distal right common femoral artery at the femoral head. The deep and superficial femoral arteries are superimposed in this projection, but you can identify the deep femoral artery because it branches. There is a large collection of extravascular contrast material with a second, less well-defined collection distally. Obviously, Mr. A. G. is still bleeding and has a pseudoaneurysm.

By this time your hands are shaking from compressing arteries, so you call in assistance. The left common femoral artery stops bleeding after 10 minutes of compression, but it takes nearly an hour to gain control on the right. Mr. A. G. is carefully observed for the next few days. He chafes at the initial bed rest, but both he and you are relieved when the swelling goes down. There is no residual mass palpable one month later, and by then Mr. A. G. has decided to have his much needed endarterectomy.

Pseudoaneurysms are one manifestation of vascular trauma. They may be of either arterial or venous origin and may be either blind pouches or conduits between two vessels. An acute pseudoaneurysm may resolve with conservative care, but those of longer duration frequently need surgical repair.

Angiography is a known cause of pseudoaneurysm, though this complication is rare. It most often occurs in debilitated patients and in those who form a large hematoma at the time of catheterization. It is not clear why Mr. A. G. developed his acute pseudoaneurysm, but both the low puncture site and the recurrent bleeding after coughing undoubtedly increased his risk.

Your troubles with Mr. A. G. remind you of Miss L. D. She was an irascible, obese, 63 year old woman with a 30 year history of diabetes. She came in for coronary angiography and possible bypass surgery. The angiogram went smoothly, and the catheter was in the right femoral artery less than 40 minutes. Miss L. D. became quite irrational when the catheter was removed and would not lie still for compression of the puncture site. Though the bleeding was eventually controlled, Miss L. D. had a hematoma measuring about 10 cm when she left the angiography suite. About one hour later, she bled again after getting out of bed against your orders. Control of the bleeding was difficult to achieve, and it was nearly an hour before you were satisfied that the hematoma, now 20 cm in diameter, was not growing. This time Miss L. D. followed your urgent instructions and remained in bed for a full six hours.

Coronary artery bypass surgery was performed without problem the next day, and Miss L. D. was ready for discharge in one week. Over this time her groin hematoma diminished in size, but there was a firm, pulsatile knot in the center of the discolored area. You request a real time ultrasound to be done prior to discharge to look for a pseudoaneurysm, but somehow Miss L. D. left the hospital without this study. Two weeks later she returns because her groin hurts, and on examination you find that the knot is now a definite mass about 6 cm in size. The groin remains discolored and is somewhat swollen. This time you escort Miss L. D. to ultrasound for a real time examination and watch the study. Real time is a dynamic procedure that must be observed or evaluated by cine, so it is hardly fair to ask you to look at this single stop frame image. It is a transverse scan over the pulsatile mass in the groin. What do you see?

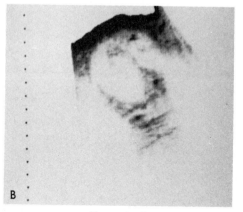

Figure 6-9b

There is a round, primarily echo-free, lesion measuring about 5 cm in greatest dimension at this level. Immediately beneath the mass is a tubular structure. Using the real time scanner in a dynamic fashion, blood could be seen swirling around in the mass. A jet of blood originated from the femoral artery and entered the mass, locating the puncture site and the neck of the pseudoaneurysm.

An angiogram was performed from the opposite groin to learn precise anatomic relationships before surgery. The results of the angiogram look much like the study on Mr. A. G. and confirm that the pseudoaneurysm arose from the superficial femoral artery. Miss L. D.

would not hold still for compression of her left groin and developed a second hematoma only slightly smaller than the first. However, she does not re-bleed and does not develop a second pseudoaneurysm. Surgical repair of the pseudoaneurysm is successful and you discharge Miss L. D., hoping she will go elsewhere if she ever needs another angiogram.

The myth that things come in threes is supported by the appearance of Ms. W. J. shortly after Mr. A. G. and Miss L. D. Miss W. J. is an eccentric young woman who got shot in the leg while trekking through the emerald mining area of Colombia. Somehow, she wandered into a restricted zone and was initially mistaken for a poacher. The guard realized she was not a thief and took her to the nearest hospital rather than to jail. In luck there, her wound was cleaned and dressed, and she was shipped to Bogotá for further care and deportation. The wound was again debrided in Bogotá but nothing else was done. When she arrives in Miami, her wound is open and ugly, but not grossly infected. Damage is mostly muscular, but she says it had bled a great deal, especially during the second debridement.

The wound granulates in time remarkably well without any infection, but about three weeks after the injury, you begin to feel a mass that seems to pulsate. Though her peripheral circulation is good, you wonder once again about a pseudoaneurysm or arteriovenous fistula. A real time ultrasound examination could be used as in Miss L. D., but W. J.'s wound is still open, making this difficult, so you order an angiogram. Two films are shown. What do you see?

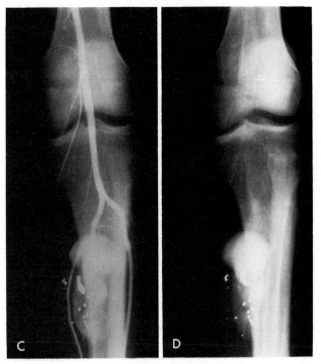

Figure 6–9c, d

The metallic bullet fragments may be the first things that catch your eye. Next you should notice that the peroneal artery empties into an irregular collection of contrast material about 1 cm distal to its origin. The posterior tibial artery is bowed medially by this collection. The later film shows no draining vein, and emptying of the sac is quite sluggish. As you suspected, W. J. has developed a post-traumatic pseudoaneurysm.

W. J. finally agrees to surgery, which is uneventful except for discovery of a venous communication that was not seen at angiography. When blood flow is very sluggish, adequate mixing of contrast medium and blood may not occur, which is the probable explanation for nonvisualization of the draining vein.

It takes W. J. some weeks to recover, and eventually skin grafting is required. In the end, she is fine and you hear from her mother that she has gone to Patagonia to try her luck again.

W. H.

W. H. is a 19 year old man who is prone to trouble. This time he has been shot in the thigh by a friend. It seems they were trying a variant of a knife throwing act using a pistol. W. H. is rather defiant when you express some surprise at this activity and says that they have been playing the game for days without trouble. In any case, he has an entry wound that is oozing blood, a rather swollen thigh and no exit wound. You can feel a femoral pulse but no distal pulses. His foot, however, is not cold or cyanotic. X-rays of the proximal femur show that the bullet lies up against the bone, but there is no bony injury. W. H. is observed in the emergency room for several hours. His peripheral pulses do not return, and the swelling continues to increase until his injured thigh is about twice as large as the other. A vascular consultant raises the question of an injury to the superficial femoral artery, which should be repaired, so an angiogram is performed. A single film is demonstrated. There are both obvious and subtle abnormalities. What are your observations?

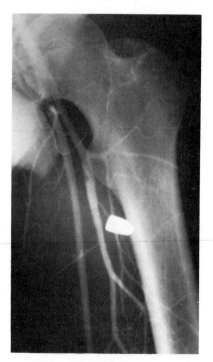

Figure 6–10

The bullet is the most obvious abnormality. You already know its location from the earlier x-rays. The superficial femoral artery has no irregularities in its lumen or evidence of disruption. The deep femoral artery, however, is abnormal. Immediately below the lesser trochanter there is a rounded filling defect. This is probably a small clot at the origin of a small transected arterial branch. Immediately lateral to this (and not to be confused with the margin of the lesser trochanter) is a fine, lucent line. This is an intimal flap or small dissection, which can be seen with blast injuries. In addition, one of the most distal branches of the deep femoral artery has a very straight course that is not anatomical. It is being stretched by the blood that has accumulated in the adjacent tissues.

W. H. is relieved when you tell him he doesn't need an immediate operation but annoyed when you tell him there can still be delayed complications. You manage to keep him in the hospital for 24 hours, by which time his peripheral pulses have returned and his thigh is less tense.

W. H. does well, or at least you don't see him again for this injury. You suspect you will see him for another in the near future.

L. H.

L. H. was working the late shift at his gas station and it was nearly closing time, so he was put out when a car pulled in. He hurried out to the car only to be confronted by a gun and a demand for gas and cash. He complied with both demands, but as he returned the nozzle to its holder, he was shot in the right arm at quite close range. The car roared off, and L. H. managed to activate a silent alarm before fainting. When the police find him, an ambulance is summoned and you are called to see L. H. when he arrives at the emergency room a few minutes later. His right arm is shattered just above the elbow. There is extensive soft tissue injury, and bone fragments can be seen on the wound. The distal arm is cool, and no pulses are palpable distal to the axilla. There is bleeding, which seems to be venous, since it stops with compression of the upper arm.

X-rays of the arm are taken. The distal third of the humerus is shattered, though the articular surfaces are spared and the elbow has a normal alignment. A myriad of small to moderate-sized bullet fragments remain around the fractured humerus. The orthopedic consultant concurs in your plan for immediate open reduction of the fracture to be done in conjunction with soft tissue debridement and repair. He is concerned about injury to the brachial artery, since the vascular status of the arm could affect the repair; and so an angiogram is requested. The study is performed from the right femoral artery. The catheter tip is placed in the distal right subclavian artery. One film from the series taken just after the contrast medium injection is illustrated. What observations can you make?

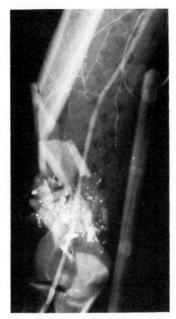

Figure 6–11

The arm is in a splint. The comminuted fracture and innumerable metallic fragments are both obvious and awful. The brachial artery is seen from its beginning to below the elbow. It has a somewhat irregular lumen compatible with spasm or compression, but there are no intraluminal filling defects, and no extravasation of contrast material is seen on this or later films. No early venous filling is present. Several small arterial branches also have luminal irregularities, and some seem to be discontinuous and others to arise from the brachial artery at an abnormal angle.

The surgical team works on the arm for several hours. L. H. has a prolonged postoperative course because of soft tissue infection, but he does not develop osteomyelitis and has use of his elbow. His right arm, however, is some inches shorter than the left when he is finally discharged.

It is not uncommon for hemorrhage and swelling around a fracture to diminish or obliterate pulses distal to the injury. The anterior compartment syndrome, which occurs with fractures of the lower leg, is another good example of this problem. It is often important to know that there is vascular integrity before tackling these fractures. Angiography can do this, though it may be necessary to use a vasodilator such as tolazoline or papaverine to relax vascular spasm. Filming over an extended period of time is also useful in making sure the entire vascular distribution has been adequately studied.

It is also important to recognize that even when you demonstrate an intact artery, such as in L. H., you have not excluded the possibility of a late complication such as pseudoaneurysm at the site of an avulsed branch or an A-V fistula that is initially compressed by the swelling. Intimal dissections can also be present and not seen. Even with these limitations, it is useful to perform angiography in cases with question of acute vascular injury, since the majority of serious injuries will be demonstrated.

CASE 6–12:

MADAME E. W.

Madame E. W. is a retired Wagnerian soprano who is one of your most trying patients. Still very much the prima donna at age 70, she is obese, diabetic and frequently irrational. Though her housekeeper tries to keep her properly fed and medicated, it is an uphill struggle and you are resigned to listening to her many complaints on your innumerable house calls. This time when the housekeeper phones, there does seem to be a serious problem. Madame has fallen, and her right leg is crumpled beneath her. She won't move and is moaning in pain. When you and the ambulance crew arrive, you find her lying at the foot of a short flight of stairs that she had forgotten. With great difficulty the three of you manage to get her onto a stretcher so you can have a look at her right leg. The most disturbing finding is the bluish cast of her lower leg. The leg is swollen from above the knee and is quite cool. She cannot fully extend her knee, and you suspect a fracture of the knee.

When you all reach the emergency room, x-rays of the knee demonstrate a depressed fracture of the medial half of the tibial plateau. Madame E. W.'s leg is still cold and blue, and so you call in orthopedic and vascular consultants. Both agree that the integrity of the popliteal artery is vital to treatment decisions, since if it is torn or occluded, loss of the lower leg would be likely in this elderly, obese woman. Acute popliteal artery injuries have a poor prognosis in the best of circumstances, and Madame E. W.'s age and condition are against her.

Madame E. W. is as reluctant to have an angiogram as the angiographer is to take it when he sees her enormous bulk. However, both recognize the importance of the study and so it is done. A preliminary film for the angiogram and two films during the film series are presented. The angiographic films were taken at six and 24 seconds after the start of the contrast medium injection. What are your observations?

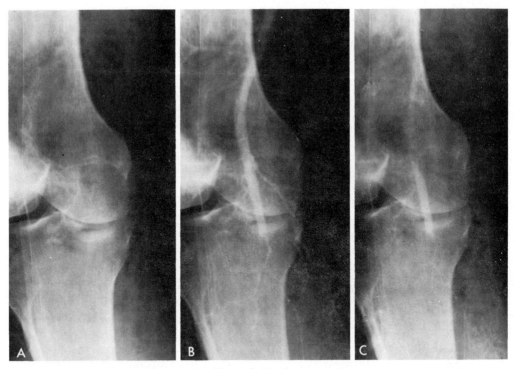

Figure 6-12a, b, c

The preliminary film shows the marked soft tissue swelling medial to the knee. The depressed medial tibial plateau fracture is also evident. The six second film shows the contrast column in the proximal popliteal artery. The artery abruptly terminates at the joint, and only a few small geniculate arteries run distally. The 24 second film shows no advance of the contrast medium column in the popliteal artery, though there has been proximal washout.

An angiographic run made after injection of papaverine, a vasodilator, does not show more distal filling of the popliteal artery. At this point you are certain that the popliteal artery is occluded. You do not know if it is occluded because of intimal damage, or is lacerated or even transected. A torn artery often goes into spasm and clots, so that a pseudoaneurysm or actual extravasation may not be seen.

The appropriate therapy for Madame E. W. is not easy to determine at this junction, but she solves your dilemma by demanding an attempt at arterial repair before any consideration of amputation. She realizes the odds of success are quite low. At surgery, there is extensive thrombosis and damage to the arterial wall without actual laceration. The vascular surgeon removes as much clot as possible and establishes a graft that is patent at the conclusion of surgery, but he holds out little hope for long-term success. The graft does occlude within a day, and Madame undergoes an amputation above the knee. She actually takes it rather well and is discharged in two weeks. She has a wheelchair custom-made for her size and even appears at an opera gala during the winter.

Popliteal artery injuries are often associated with rotatory injuries to the knee. Repair is difficult, and even in the young, collateral circulation may not be adequate to sustain the limb. Early diagnosis by arteriography is mandatory in the evaluation of such a patient.

Y. C.

The annual family reunion is in full swing with 38 adults and about 70 children all enjoying themselves in both sedentary and athletic pursuits when a loud clatter of shattering glass followed by a child screaming occurs. Y. C. has run through a plate glass window and is covered with blood, most of which is coming from his left arm. All the first aid experts gather around, and someone presses on Y. C.'s upper arm, effectively stopping the bleeding. His father and a cousin bring Y. C. into the emergency room.

Examination reveals that Y. C. is really more scared than hurt, but he does have a nasty laceration on his upper arm that bleeds copiously whenever pressure is released. Pulses are not palpable distal to the laceration, but the arm is warm. You are concerned about an arterial injury and, after discussion with his father, decide to request an angiogram. Two films of the angiogram are demonstrated. The first is at two seconds after the start of the contrast medium injection, and the second is five seconds later. What do you think?

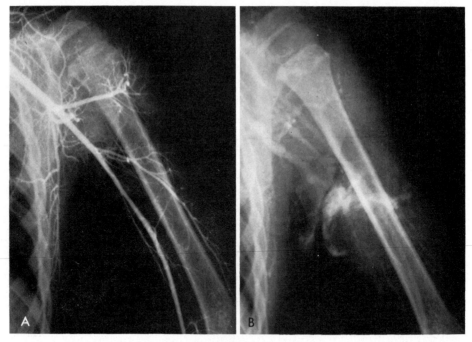

Figure 6–13a, b

The arterial phase is almost normal, though there is some narrowing of the brachial artery, probably because of spasm. The interesting observation is on the second film taken during the venous phase. There is marked extravasation of contrast material on this film. The timing of the extravasation tells you the bleeding is venous. Prolonged direct compression finally stops the bleeding and the laceration is sutured. Y. C. goes home the next day with all kinds of gory tales to tell.

As you reflect on the case of H. S., you are not sure whether it should be considered traumatic or historical in nature. H. S. is a 56 year old man who left a successful career in the stock market about 10 years ago. Brought low by alcohol, he has become a rider of the rails, occasionally seeking odd jobs. You were his physician in his affluent days and are surprised and dismayed by what you see when he drops by one afternoon. He has gangrene of several toes and one fingertip and complains of incredible burning in his arms and legs. You can feel no peripheral pulses, though he has palpable axillary, carotid and femoral pulses. It is summer, so he can't have a frostbite, and he has had no untoward contact with electricity or other physical trauma.

The picture is confusing, and you inquire about his current living arrangements. He denies all drugs other than alcohol and looks rather well nourished. In fact, he tells you he found some discarded grain recently, which he has been grinding and using for porridge and a flat bread he makes in a frying pan. An idea comes to mind and grows stronger when you learn that the grain is indeed rye. You admit H. S. to the hospital and schedule angiography of his extremities along with a vascular surgical consultation. Angiography is performed the next day. What are you looking for? Do you find it?

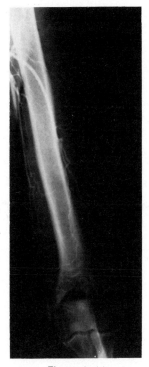

Figure 6–14

A single late arterial film from a left subclavian arterial injection is shown. The axillary artery tapers off rapidly and appears to be occluded. Only rather small, collateral arteries are seen reaching the elbow. The findings are those of ergotism caused, in this case, by a fungus infection of the rye grain. Though the areas of gangrene will not return to normal, most of the vascular spasm will reverse when the source of ergot is removed. H. S. gets away with loss of several toes and one fingertip. Slightly wiser, he considers re-entering the business world, but the feel of a shirt and tie convinces him to return to his roving life.

Ergotism, once known as St. Anthony's fire or Holy Fire, is now a rare condition, seen infrequently in patients taking ergot for relief of migraine headaches. The disease results in profound arterial spasm with superimposed thrombosis. The spasm is reversible, but areas of gangrene are not.

INDEX

Note: Page numbers in *italics* refer to illustrations.